SOUL OF APPALACHIA

A HILLBILLY COOKBOOK

KIMBERLEY RUSSELL

HOPE RUSSELL

GILDED PAGE PUBLISHING

INTRODUCTION

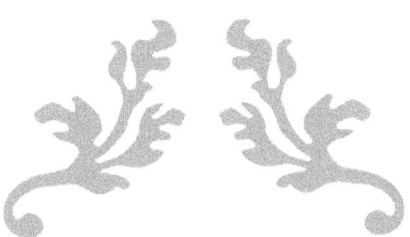

The Soul of Appalachia a Hillbilly cookbook, by Kimberley Russell and Hope Russell
A family collection of old favorite recipes from historical eras like the WW2 era, plus new variations like cornbread without flour, and some other invented at home unique recipes. It is important to note that copyright for recipe books is more to cover the collection or arrangement of the recipes than the individual recipes themselves.

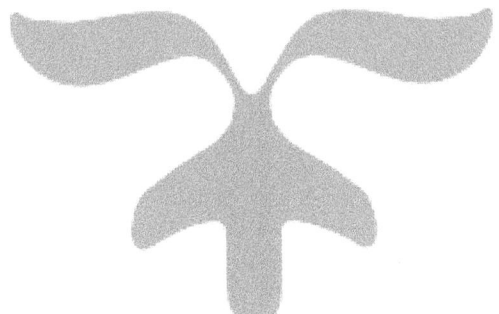

2

BREADS

B reads:

AND JESUS SAID UNTO THEM, i am the bread of life: he that cometh to me shall never hunger; and he that believeth on me shall never thirst. john 6:35

KIMMY'S SOUTHERN CORNBREAD

Kimmy's Southern cornbread
SHOPPING LIST
cornmeal
eggs
butter
olive oil
Milk
Bacon for drippings

Variations: If you have egg allergies you can substitute sour cream for the egg, use 2T sour cream per egg. If you love eggs and want a stronger bread you can use 2 eggs instead of the 1 I use. You can crumble the bacon into the bread for "crackle bread".

Servings | Prep Time | Total Time

Ingredients

2 cups cornmeal

1 egg

1 stick butter, melted

¼ cup olive oil

Milk add till cornbread is runny

Bacon to fry for drippings

Directions

Dump the cornmeal in a large bowl, add the egg, the oil and the melted butter. Add the milk while stirring a bit at a time till the mix is runny. You want it thinner than a cake would be. If you are cooking the corn bread in a cast iron pan, add butter or bacon drippings to the pan and heat it in the oven at 350F till hot, pour in the cornbread mix and it will sizzle, this makes a yummy crust on the outside of the bread. Bake the bread in the oven at 350F till the top is golden brown and a knife inserted comes out clean. Normally this is about 30-40 minutes, the resulting time will vary in different humidity locations.

4

PLAIN BISCUITS

Plain Biscuits
    2 cups sifted flour
    4 tsp baking powder
1 tsp salt
3 T powdered milk
1/3 cup shortening, or a stick of butter, grated
¾ cup water

Sift the dry ingredients together into a large bowl. Work the shortening into the mix with a pastry blender or fork. Stir in the water to form a soft dough. Turn the dough out onto a floured surface and knead 10 times. Roll out to ½ inch thickness and cut out biscuits with a glass or a cookie cutter. Flour the cutter to keep it from sticking to the dough. Bake in the oven for 12 minutes at 425F Make sure the pan was greased before adding the biscuits. Biscuits should be golden brown, tan really.

BANANA NUT BREAD

B anana Nut Bread
2 cups flour
3 ½ tsp baking powder
½ tsp salt
½ cup chopped pecans or other type nuts
1 egg beaten, or 2 T yogurt
3 medium overripe bananas, squished up
¼ cup milk
½ cup sour cream
1/3 cup melted butter

Mix all the ingredients quickly, but completely. Pour the mixture into a greased and floured loaf pan. Bake at 350F for 45-50 minutes. Insert a knife to check for doneness. The knife should come out mostly clean. The bread will pull away from the sides of the pan a bit. Let cool for at least 5 minutes before placing a tray over the pan and flipping it to turn out the loaf for easy slicing. Let the bread cool before slicing.

ORANGE NUT BREAD

O range Nut Bread
    2 T softened butter
    1 cup honey
1 egg (if anyone has egg allergies use 2 T plain yogurt instead)
1 T grated orange rind
2 ¾ cups flour
2 ½ tsp baking powder
½ tsp baking soda
½ tsp salt
¾ cup orange juice
¾ cup chopped pecans, or any nut you like
1 tsp orange flavoring
Orange cream glaze
1 3oz package of cream cheese
¼ cup orange juice
½ tsp grated orange peel
½ T sugar

For the bread, Blend the softened butter and honey together. Beat the egg and add the orange rind, mix well. Sift the dry ingredients together and add to the egg mixture, alternating with the orange juice. Mix in the nuts. Pour the mixture into a greased loaf pan and bake at 350F for 45minutes to an hour, till a knife inserted comes out clean.

. . .

BLEND THE CREAM CHEESE, that has sat out to soften before you started, with the orange juice and peel and sugar, for your glaze. Pour over top of the hot bread when it comes out of the oven. You can poke holes in the bread to allow the glaze to penetrate the bread topmost layers.

MIXED WHEAT SOURDOUGH TYPE BREAD

Mixed wheat Sourdough Bread
You will keep starter in the refrigerator, and it needs to be "fed" every 3-5 days. The 'feed' is 1 1/3 cup of sugar, 6 T potato flakes, 2 2/3 cups warm water. The actual starter is 1 pkg. regular yeast, 1 cup warm water, ¾ cup sugar, 3 T instant potato flakes. Combine the ingredients of the starter, don't bloom the yeast just mix it in. Let it sit on the counter for 5 hours to ferment. Refrigerate for 3-5 days in a glass jar before using it and feed it every 3-5 days to keep it ready for bread making.

When you are ready to make bread, you will be using the starter that hasn't been fed for at least 3 days. You will leave the starter on the counter before using it for 8-12 hours, till it is bubbly. Stir well before use.

Bread:

In a large bowl, you will be making a stiff dough:

1/3 cup sugar

4 cups bread flour, 3 cups whole wheat flour

2 cups of starter

½ cup corn oil

1 cup water

1 tsp salt

Feed the remaining starter as usual and return it to the refrigerator to use on future breads. Remember to feed it every 3-5 days.

Oil the inside of a large bowl, put the dough in the bowl, and oil the top of the dough. Cover the dough with a towel and let it sit overnight at room temperature.

The next morning punch down the dough and divide it into 3 equal parts. Knead each part until no more air bubbles are present, then put each part into an oiled loaf pan, press down the dough until it covers the bottom of the pan. Oil the top of each loaf and cover the pans with a towel. Let rise (5-6 hours in summer, all day in winter). Bake at 325-350F for 30-35 minutes. Remove from pans immediately, brush the tops with butter, and cool on a wire rack.

IF YOU WANT a cinnamon version of this bread add 2 T cinnamon to the stiff dough ingredients. You can let butter soften on the counter and whip it with cinnamon and honey too as a spread for the bread. Keep the butter spread refrigerated when not in use.

EASY BREAD

Easy bread
   3 cups all-purpose flour
   2 T instant yeast
1 tsp salt
1 cup warm water
2 T olive oil
2 T butter, melted to brush on top
Pinch of sugar

In a large mixing bowl, combine the flour, sugar, instant yeast and salt. Mix well. Gradually add the warm water and olive oil stirring with a wooden spoon, or your hands till a dough forms. Tun the dough onto a floured surface and knead 8-10 minutes, till it becomes smooth and elastic. If its too sticky add flour 1 T at a time. Place the kneaded dough in a lightly greased bowl, cover with a clean kitchen towel and let rise in a warm place for 1 hour, or until it doubles in size. Punch it down to release the air. Divide the dough into 6-8 pieces. Shape each piece into a ball, flatten it slightly to form a disc. It should be around ½ inch thick. Heat a heavy cast iron skillet over medium low heat, don't grease it. Place the disks in the skillet, but not touching each other. Cover with a lid. Cook 5-7 minutes on each side till golden brown. Bread will fluff up as it cooks. Brush with butter and serve.

CHOCOLATE ORANGE NUT BREAD

Chocolate orange Nut Bread
  2 T softened butter
  1 cup honey
1 egg (if anyone has egg allergies use 2 T plain yogurt instead)
1 T grated orange rind
2 ¾ cups flour
2 ½ tsp baking powder
½ tsp baking soda
½ tsp salt
¼ cup cocoa
¾ cup orange juice
¾ cup chopped pecans, or any nut you like
1 tsp orange flavoring
Chocolate Orange cream glaze
1 3oz package of cream cheese
3 T orange juice
½ tsp grated orange peel
1 square semi-sweet baking chocolate, melted
½ T sugar

For the bread, Blend the softened butter and honey together. Beat the egg and add the orange rind, mix well. Sift the dry ingredients together and add to the egg mixture, alternating with the orange juice. Mix in the nuts. Pour the mixture into a greased loaf pan and bake at 350F for 45minutes to an hour, till a knife inserted comes out clean.

BLEND THE CREAM CHEESE, that has sat out to soften before you started, with the orange juice, chocolate, orange peel and sugar, for your glaze. Pour over top of the hot bread when it comes out of the oven. You can poke holes in the bread to allow the glaze to penetrate the bread topmost layers.

BISHOP'S BREAD

Bishop's Bread
    2 cups sugar
    1 ¾ cups flour
¾ cup dark chocolate cocoa
1 ½ tsp baking powder
1 ½ tsp baking soda
½ tsp salt
2 eggs
1 cup sour cream
½ cup butter, melted
2 T rum
1 cup boiling water
1 pkg semi-sweet chocolate chips
1 jar maraschino cherries, chopped
1 pkg butterscotch chips
1 cup pecans, chopped

Preheat the oven to 350F. Grease and flour 2 loaf pans. Stir together the sugar, flour, cocoa, baking powder, baking soda and salt in a large bowl. Add the eggs, sour cream, butter and rum. Beat with mixer on medium speed for 2 minutes. Stir in the boiling water the batter will be needing to cool a bit. Mix the chocolate chips, cherries and butterscotch chips and nuts together in a bowl and dust with ¼ cup flour. Mix to coat all the pieces. Fold into the cake batter, blend then pour the cakes in the loaf pans. Bake at 350F for 35-40 minutes, or till a toothpick inserted comes out mostly clear of crumbs. You will see some melted candy, but that's normal. You don't want cake batter to stick.

ORANGE Scones

    2 cups sifted flour

    3 tsp baking powder

    ½ tsp salt

    3 T sugar

    6 T butter

    ¼ cup evaporated milk

    2 T orange juice

    2 eggs

    Orange marmalade

    Granulated sugar

Sift together the flour, baking powder, salt and sugar. Cut in the butter with a pastry cutter or two knives. Combine the milk and orange juice. Beat the eggs well and combine with the milk mixture. Add the milk mixture to the dry ingredients a bit at a time, only enough to moisten. Turn out the dough onto a floured surface and lightly roll it to ¼ inch thick. Cut into 1 ½ inch squares. Spread the orange marmalade on ½ the squares, then top the marmalade squares with the plain ones. Seal the edges lightly and sprinkle the tops with the granulated sugar. You can add orange zest to the sugar as well. Or you can make a fast glaze with orange juice 2 T water and some powdered sugar and orange zest, to use on the cooked scones. Place the scones on a greased cookie sheet to bake at 400F for 12-15 minutes. If using glaze top them while hot.

11

BUTTER PECAN BREAD

Butter Pecan bread
1/3 cup butter
1 cup dark brown sugar

2 eggs

2 ½ cups flour, sifted

2 tsp baking powder

½ tsp salt

½ tsp cinnamon

½ tsp baking soda

1 cup buttermilk

1 ½ cup pecans, chopped

2 T caramel flavoring

2 tsp butter extract or butterscotch flavoring

In a mixing bowl cream, the butter and sugar, beat in the eggs, one at a time. Sift together the flour, baking powder, salt, cinnamon, and baking soda. Add the sifted ingredients alternating with the buttermilk. Add the pecans and flavorings, blend. Pour the mixture into a buttered loaf pan. Bake at 325F 50 minutes. Turn out onto a wire rack to cool.

12

WHOLE WHEAT BREAD

Whole Wheat bread
1 pkg dry yeast
2 cups warm water
3 T oil
3 T molasses, or honey
4 cups whole wheat flour
1 cup wheat germ
1 ½ cup powdered milk
1 tsp salt
½ tsp cinnamon

Stir the dry yeast into the warm water. Into the mixture, stir the oil and molasses or honey. Add 3 cups of the flour, stir 300 strokes by hand or until smooth. Add the wheat germ, the remaining flour, the milk and the salt and cinnamon. Mix well, you want all the ingredients moistened. Cover the bowl, set in a warm place to allow it to rise to double its size. This is an hour in the summer, maybe longer in the winter. Pour the bread out onto a floured surface to knead. Make it mixed well, and flexible, should feel kind of like an earlobe in softness. Divide it into 2 loaves. Oil 2 loaf pans and put the loaves in the pan, working it to cover the bottom of the pans. Oil the tops of the loaves, lightly. Cover the pans with a towel and let rise again till double in size. Bake in a preheated oven at 325F for 45 minutes. Don't overbake, or the bread will be dry.

13

CARROT NUT BREAD

Carrot Nut Bread

    3 eggs, if you have egg sensitivity use ½ cup yogurt instead

    1 ½ cups sugar

1 cup butter, melted

1 cup whole wheat flour

1 ¼ cup regular flour

1 ¼ tsp baking soda

1 ½ tsp cinnamon

1 tsp ginger

½ tsp nutmeg

½ tsp salt

2 ¼ cups finely grated carrots

1 ½ cup pecans, chopped

1 ¼ cup chopped dates

1 tsp rum

½ cup sour cream

Beat the eggs well. Add the sugar and butter and beat till light. Mix the flours, soda, cinnamon, ginger, nutmeg, salt, add them to the egg mixture and stir just till everything is well moistened. Stir in the rest of the ingredients and pour it into the well-greased loaf pan. Bake at 350F for 1 ½ hours or till a knife comes out clean. Cool in the pan 10 minutes before trying to remove from the pan.

14

BLUEBERRY MUFFINS

Blueberry Muffins
  1 egg
  ¾ cup buttermilk
1/3 cup butter, melted
3 large spoonfuls sour cream
1 ½ cup flour
¼ cup sugar
2 ½ cup baking powder
½ tsp salt
1 cup pecans, chopped
1 ½ cup wild blueberries
1 tsp blueberry juice (you can make it by covering some blueberries with sugar and leaving them to make the juice overnight in the refrigerator).
1 tsp almond flavoring

Combine the egg, buttermilk and butter, mix well. Sift together the dry ingredients and add them, gently mixing. Fold in the nuts, berries, juice and flavoring. Fill greased muffin tins 2/3 of the way full. Bake at 350F for 25 minutes.

PEANUT BUTTER MAPLE MUFFINS

Peanut Butter maple muffins
Sift together:
2 cups flour
3 tsp baking powder
½ tsp salt
½ cup sugar
1 tsp maple flavoring
Add:
¾ cup peanut butter
2 T butter, melted

Work the peanut butter and butter into the flour with a fork. It will be crumbly. Mix in:

1 egg
1 cup milk

Mixing lightly. Don't over-mix. Fill the muffin tin ½ full or you can bake this as a bread in a loaf pan. Grease the pan either way. Bake at 350F for 20-25 minutes till browned.

16

DOUGHNUTS

Doughnuts
    Sift together 3 times:
    4 cups flour
1 tsp baking soda
½ tsp salt
½ tsp cinnamon
¼ tsp nutmeg
1 cup sugar
Combine in a mixing bowl:
2 eggs, slightly beaten
1 cup buttermilk
Add the sifted ingredients all at once, just dump it in. stir till just blended, don't over-mix.
    Stir in:
    2 T butter, melted
Chill. When ready to make, cut out circles with a cookie cutter, cut the whole out with a small bottle cap. Fry in a deep fryer in fat. Immediately cover in powdered sugar or cinnamon sugar.

DINNER ROLLS

Dinner rolls
     2 cups milk
     ½ cup butter, soft
¼ cup sugar
Boil the above and set aside to cool to lukewarm.
Combine:
1 pkg. yeast
½ cup lukewarm water
Sift together:
7 cups flour
1 tsp baking soda
½ tsp salt
1 tsp baking powder
Combine the yeast mixture and the milk mixture. Blend the combined milk mixture into the dry ingredients till well mixed. Store overnight in the fridge, covered. When ready to make take small amounts of dough, hand form the dough rolls, put them to rise to double the size. Bake at 400F for 12-14 minutes. Makes 70 rolls.

BLACK WALNUT COCONUT BREAD

B lack Walnut coconut bread
      Beat until light:
      3 eggs
Stir in:
½ cup butter, melted
3 T black walnut flavoring
Add:
2 cups shredded coconut
1 ½ cups black walnuts, chopped
1 cup chopped dates
½ cup sour cream
Sift together and stir in till just blended:
2 cups flour
½ tsp salt
1 tsp baking soda
1 tsp baking powder
1 tsp cinnamon
1 cup sugar
Pour into a well-greased loaf pan, bake at 350F for 1 hour or until it tests done. Start testing at 45 minutes.

SIMPLE BREAD

Simple bread
Dissolve:
1 pkg. dry active yeast in
½ cup warm water
Dissolve:
1 ½ tsp salt and 3 T sugar in:
1 cup hot milk
When the milk mixture is lukewarm add the yeast mixture.
Add:
3 T corn oil
Blend in:
4 cups flour
Knead till smooth and elastic. It should feel kind of like an earlobe. Place the dough in an oiled bowl, turn the dough to oil all sides. Cover with a towel and put in a warm place to rise to double its size. Punch it down to remove air. Split into 2 halves. Oil 2 loaf pans, and put the bread into the pans, covering the whole bottom. Cover with a towel and let it rise to double again. Brush the tops with oil. Slash across the top with a knife, in a few places. Bake at 375F till golden brown. Should be around 50 minutes.

ONE DAY DINNER ROLLS

O ne day dinner rolls

        1 pkg. dry active yeast

        ½ cup lukewarm water

1 ½ tsp salt

2 large T sugar

1 ½ cups butter, soft

¾ cups hot water

1 egg, beaten

4 cups flour, plus 1 cup to work in

Dissolve the yeast in the lukewarm water. In a mixing bowl, put butter, sugar and salt. Pour the hot water over this. When it cools to lukewarm add the yeast mixture. Add beaten egg and flour 1 cup at a time, beat after each cup. After mixing well, chill in the refrigerator for 1 hour. Shape into rolls, place on the baking sheet, cover with a towel and let rise to double size. Bake at 400F for 20 minutes till browned.

BANANA BLACK WALNUT BREAD

Banana Black Walnut bread
¾ cup butter, soft
4 bananas, overripe, mashed
1 tsp vanilla
3 T black walnut flavoring
1 tsp baking soda
1/8 cup buttermilk
1 ½ cups sugar
2 eggs, well beaten
1 1/3 cups whole wheat flour
2/3 cups rolled oats
1 cup black walnuts, chopped

Cream the butter and sugar well. Blend in the bananas, eggs and flavorings. Sift the flour, soda and salt together. Add the oats, mix well. Stir the flour mixture into the banana mixture gradually, alternating with the milk. Add the nuts, mix well. Pour into a greased and floured loaf pan. Bake at 325F for 1 hour or till done. Let it sit in the pan for 30 minutes before trying to remove it from the pan. Be sure to bake on the bottom shelf of the oven.

CRANBERRY ORANGE BREAD

Cranberry Orange bread
Combine in a mixing bowl:
2 cups self-rising flour
1 cup sugar
½ tsp baking soda
½ tsp salt
Add:
1 egg
2 T melted butter
2 T hot cranberry juice
½ cup orange juice
½ tsp orange flavoring
Stir in:
1 cup pecans, chopped
1 cup cranberries, frozen, chopped and thawed
Pour into a greased and floured loaf pan. Bake at 350F for 1 hour or till done.

LEMON BLUEBERRY BREAD

L emon blueberry bread
Cream together:
¾ cup sugar
2 eggs
3 T butter, soft
Sift together:
2 ¼ cups all-purpose flour
3 tsp baking powder
½ tsp salt
Add the dry ingredients alternately with:
½ cup buttermilk
Blend well. Stir in:
1 cup pecans, chopped
1 cup wild blueberries
2 tsp. grated lemon zest
2 T lemon juice

Pour into greased and floured loaf pan and bake at 350F for 55-60 minutes. If using self-rising flour, leave out the baking powder and salt. Except in cases where the flour might not be good at rising, like if it's near the expiration date, if it's close to expiration use the baking powder and salt.

24

SUN-DRIED TOMATO AND PROVOLONE CHEESE BREAD

Sun-dried tomato and provolone bread
    1/3 cup oil packed sun-dried tomatoes
    2 ¼ cup flour
2 tsp baking powder
1 tsp sugar
1 ¼ tsp dried basil
½ tsp rosemary
½ tsp salt
½ tsp baking soda
½ tsp black pepper
2 eggs or if allergic ¼ cup sour cream
1 ¼ cups buttermilk
3 T olive oil
1 cup shredded provolone
¼ cup chopped fine parsley

Preheat the oven to 350F. Drain the tomatoes, reserving the oil. Chop the tomatoes and set aside. In a large bowl combine the flour, baking powder, sugar, basil, rosemary, salt baking soda, and pepper. In a small bowl whisk the egg, buttermilk, olive oil, and 2 T of the tomato oil. Stir in the dry ingredients till just moistened. Fold in the cheese, parsley and sun-dried tomatoes. Split the dough into thirds and put 1 of each in a greased small loaf pan. Bake 40-45 minutes or until a toothpick inserted comes out clean. Cool 10 minutes in the pan before removing. Cool on wire racks.

CHEESECAKE FACTORY COPYCAT BROWN BREAD

Cheesecake Factory copycat brown bread
2 ½ cups warm water
2 ½ tsp active dry yeast
2 T sugar
3 cups whole wheat flour
3 T cocoa powder
2 tsp instant coffee powder
1 tsp salt
¼ cup honey
¼ cup molasses
¼ cup butter, melted
3-4 cups bread flour
Cooking spray
Cornmeal for dusting, or rolled oats

In the body of a stand mixer with the dough hook add the warm water, yeast and sugar, stir a few times to combine. Let sit for 5 minutes till its bubbly. While waiting, stir together the flour, cocoa, coffee and salt set aside. Once the yeast is bubbly, add the honey, molasses, and melted butter, stir to combine. Add the dry ingredients to the wet mixture, stir and scrape sides to incorporate it all. Add the 2 ½ cups bread flour and stir till combined. At low speed add a little bread flour at a time till dough comes off the sides of the bowl. Turn the speed up to knead it on medium high for 6-7 minutes. If it sticks to the sides of the bowl add a bit more bread flour. Spray a large bowl with cooking spray. Add the dough and oil the top of the bread with olive oil. Cover with a kitchen towel and let rise to double the size. 45-90 minutes in a warm kitchen. Punch down the dough to remove air bubbles. On a lightly floured surface, divide the dough in 4 equal loaves. Place them into loaf pans and press down lightly to cover the bottom. Oil the tops of the loaves and sprinkle with the cornmeal or oats. Cover with a towel and let rise again. 30 minutes in a warm kitchen. They should double in size. Heat the oven to 350F. bake for 20-25 minutes, till the bread is no longer shiny, and it should start looking crusty. The internal temperature needs to be 200-210F. let it cool before slicing.

KIMMY'S SOUTHERN CORNBREAD PANCAKES

Kimmy's southern cornbread pancakes
SHOPPING LIST
cornmeal
eggs
butter
olive oil
Milk
Bacon for drippings

Variations: If you have egg allergies you can substitute sour cream for the egg, use 2T sour cream per egg. If you love eggs and want a stronger bread you can use 2 eggs instead of the 1 I use. You can crumble the bacon into the bread for "crackle bread".

Servings | Prep Time | Total Time

Ingredients

2 cups cornmeal

1 egg

1 stick butter, melted

¼ cup olive oil

Milk add till cornbread is runny

Bacon to fry for drippings

Directions

Dump the cornmeal in a large bowl, add the egg, the oil and the melted butter. Add the milk while stirring a bit at a time till the mix is runny. You want it thinner than a cake would be, especially for pancakes. The runnier the mix the thinner the pancake. Let each side set up and turn golden brown before flipping and mash the pancake down flatter if thin pancakes are your goal. The thin ones are crispy, the thicker ones will be not crispy and more like traditional pancake texture. We use honey on ours if we want them sweet.

CHOCOLATE BANANA NUT BREAD

Chocolate banana nut bread
      1 tsp baking soda
      ¼ cup water (warm)
1 cup butter, soft
1 1/3 cup sugar
2 eggs
3 overripe bananas, mashed
2 cups flour
1/3 cup cocoa
1 tsp vanilla
1 cup pecans, chopped

Grease and flour a 9X5 loaf pan, set it aside. Combine the baking soda and warm water and set it aside. Cream the butter and add the sugar and beat till light and fluffy. Add the eggs one at a time beating in between. Beat in the bananas at low speed, add the flour, cocoa and soda water mix. Add the vanilla and beat till blended. Fold in the nuts. Bake at 350F for an hour. A toothpick inserted should come out clean.

28

PIZZA DOUGH

Pizza dough
>2 tsp powdered active yeast
>1/3 cup plus 2T warm water

1 ½ cups flour

4T olive oil

½ tsp salt

Dissolve the yeast in the warm water, completely. Mix all the ingredients together in a large bowl. Knead like crazy for 5 minutes on a heavily floured board till your fingers hurt. Put the dough in a clean lightly oiled bowl. Cover with a kitchen towel in a warm place. Allow the dough to rise for an hour in a warm kitchen. It should be twice its original size. Knead a bit and put it into the pizza pan, be sure to grease it first. Bake at 450F for enough time to set it and see it beginning to toast. Remove from oven and build your fillings into the crust. You will bake the pizza at 400F, till the cheese is melted and the pizza hot.

29

SALT RISING BREAD

Salt rising bread
   This bread uses a starter that ferments.
   Starter:

1 cup milk

1T sugar

7T corn meal, white

1 tsp salt

Scald the milk, and stir in the sugar, corn meal and salt. Put this mixture in a clean canning jar and place the jar in a hot water bath with the lid on to ferment. Keep the water bath warm for 6-7 hours to ferment. After the 6-7 hours add:

2 cups flour

2 cups lukewarm water

2 T sugar

3 T butter, melted

Beat the two mixtures together well and return them to the jar. Put the lid on the jar and keep in a hot water bath till the mixture is light and bubbly. Now put it in a bowl and add:

8 ½ cups flour, sifted

Work the flour into the mixture to make a stiff dough. Knead 10-15 minutes and divide the dough into loaves, this is 3 ½ pounds. Place the loaves in buttered loaf pans and cover with a towel to rise. It will rise to 2 ½ times its original size. Bake at 380F for 10 minutes, then reduce the oven temperature to 350 for another 35 minutes.

30

SCOTCH SCONE BREAD

Scotch scone bread
    ½ cup sugar
    ¼ tsp salt
2 cups flour
2 tsp baking powder
½ tsp baking soda
1 stick butter, grated
Sift the dry ingredients together, work the butter in with a pastry cutter or 2 knives to make a cornmeal consistency. Add:
    2 eggs, slightly beaten
Buttermilk, enough for soft dough to form
Put the dough in a well-greased baking pan and sprinkle the top with sugar. Bake at 350F for 20 minutes. Serve hot with butter.

CREAM BISCUITS

Cream biscuits
1 cup cream
1 ½ cups flour
2 tsp baking powder
Pinch of salt

Mix together well but handle as little as possible. Turn out onto a floured board. Pat flat to ½ inch thickness. Cut out biscuits. Bake at 350-400F till golden.

WHIPPED CREAM BISCUITS

Whipped cream biscuits
   2 cups flour
   3 tsp baking powder
½ tsp salt
1 cup heavy whipping cream, whipped

Sift the dry ingredients together, twice. Add the whipping cream and gently work it in with a fork. Turn out onto a floured board. Gently knead just a bit. Roll with very light pressure to ½ inch thick. Bake at 400F 10-12 minutes till golden.

BREAKFAST FOODS

B reakfast foods

1. SOUR CREAM MUFFINS
2. ORANGE ALMOND MUFFINS
3. CINNAMON ROLLS
4. PEANUT BUTTER BISCUITS
5. BUTTERMILK ROLLS
6. APPLE PANCAKES
7. GINGERBREAD PANCAKES
8. BUTTERMILK PANCAKES
9. CREPES
10. CHOCOLATE PECAN PANCAKES
11. FUDGE SAUCE (FOR CHOCOLATE PANCAKES)

GIVE us this day our daily bread. Matthew 6:11

SOUR CREAM MUFFINS

S our cream muffins
    2 cups flour, sifted
    2 tsp baking powder
½ tsp baking soda
1 T water
2 T sugar
½ tsp salt
1 egg
1 cup sour cream

Sift the flour, baking powder and sugar into a large bowl. Beat eggs. Add the cream and baking soda mixed into the water to the dry ingredients. Add the beaten eggs. Stir only enough to moisten the batter, don't try to mash out lumps. Butter the muffin tins and fill 2/3 of the way with batter. Bake at 400F till crust is golden brown.

Variation: you can add ½ cup crushed drained pineapple or ½ cup nuts, etc. even chocolate chips would be good.

ORANGE ALMOND MUFFINS

O range almond muffins
1 ½ cups flour
2 ½ tsp baking powder
½ tsp salt
2/3 cup buttermilk
1 tsp orange zest
1 tsp orange juice
1 tsp almond flavoring
2 T melted butter
1 egg

In one bowl sift the dry ingredients together. Beat the other ingredients together in another bowl. Beat the liquids into the dry ingredients gradually add 2 more T melted butter. Fill the buttered muffin tins ½ way up and set aside. Fry some sliced almonds in a skillet till golden in 1 T butter 1 tsp brown sugar ½ tsp cinnamon and 1 tsp orange juice. Spoon this onto the muffins before baking at 400F for 12-15 minutes.

CINNAMON ROLLS

C innamon rolls
¾ cup scalded milk
¼ cup sugar

2 ½ T butter flavored Crisco 2 ½ T butter

1 tsp salt

3 packets dry active yeast, dissolved in ¼ cup lukewarm water

1 egg, beaten

3 ½ cups flour

Place the sugar, salt and Crisco/butter combo in a bowl. Pour the scalded milk over them and gently stir. Allow to cool. Beat the egg and add it to the yeast. Add the yeast mixture to the milk mixture. Add ½ cup of the flour and beat well. Add the rest of the flour and blend it in. Chill the dough for an hour in the refrigerator. After its chilled, turn it out onto a floured surface and roll out into a jelly roll rectangle. Smear the rectangle with lots of butter, sprinkle it heavily with cinnamon and brown sugar. Roll up the jelly roll and slice into the pinwheels for the cinnamon rolls. They should be ½ inch thick. In the bottom of a baking pan melt butter and brown sugar to create a base for the cinnamon pinwheels to rest on. Lay the pinwheels into this but not touching. Let rise for 2 hours. The rolls should double in size when risen. Bake 350 for 12-15 minutes. You can make a cinnamon glaze to go on top

Glaze: ¼ cup powdered sugar, 1 tsp cinnamon, 1 T orange juice, 1/8 cup water. Cook on low heat till the mixture starts to thicken, stirring constantly. When it coats a spoon pull it off the heat. Let it sit a few minutes then apply it to the warm cinnamon rolls.

PEANUT BUTTER BISCUITS

Peanut butter biscuits
  4 T peanut butter
  2 T butter
½ tsp salt
4 tsp baking powder
2 cups flour
Buttermilk

Sift the dry ingredients into a bowl. Cut in the peanut butter and butter with a pastry cutter or 2 knives. Make a well in the middle and add buttermilk, pushing in the sides till the dry mix is a soft dough. Turn out the dough onto a floured board and pat it down to ½ inch thickness. Cut out the biscuits and bake at 350F for 12-15 minutes till golden.

38

BUTTERMILK ROLLS

Buttermilk rolls
2 cups buttermilk
3 pkgs dry active yeast
2 T sugar
1 tsp salt
¼ tsp baking soda
4 cups flour
2 T butter, melted

Dissolve the yeast in ¼ cup of the buttermilk. Add the sugar, salt and baking soda to the rest of the buttermilk. Add the yeast mixture and beat in ½ the flour till its smooth and full of bubbles. Add the melted butter and mix in the rest of the flour till a stiff dough forms. Turn the dough onto a floured surface and knead till it is elastic and smooth. You want to do this quickly and lightly, don't overdo it. Roll the dough to ½ inch thick and brush on melted butter. Cut into square rolls and lay on a baking sheet. Cover with a towel and let it rise for about an hour to double the original size. Bake at 350F for 20 minutes till golden. Serve hot with butter and honey at breakfast or dinner.

39

APPLE PANCAKES

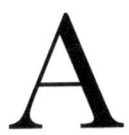pple pancakes
     1-2 tart apples, sliced
     1 tsp cinnamon
¼ cup dark brown sugar
½ stick butter
Lay the sliced apples in a baking pan and top with the remaining ingredients. Bake at 300F till the apples are soft when poked by a fork. Remove from the oven and set aside.

3 eggs, well beaten
1 cup buttermilk
½ tsp salt
2 cups flour
½ tsp baking powder
Combine the eggs, milk, salt and baking powder, mix well. Add the flour till a creamy dough forms. Add the apples and add more milk if needed. Fry on both sides till each side is golden. Wait to flip till the bottom side is golden and the edges of the pancake look dry and less shiny. Top with your favorite topping.

40

GINGERBREAD PANCAKES

Gingerbread pancakes
2 eggs
½ cup melted butter
½ cup sugar
¼ cup molasses
½ cup buttermilk
2 cups flour
½ tsp baking powder
1 tsp ginger
½ tsp cinnamon
¼ tsp nutmeg

In a bowl sift the flour, baking powder and spices together and set aside. Beat eggs till light. Add in the butter, sugar and beat again. Mix in the molasses and milk. Gradually add the flour and spice mixture. Blend well. Fry the pancakes on both sides till golden. Top with ginger cream

Ginger cream: 2 cups heavy whipping cream, beat till peaks form. Add ¼ cup sugar and 1 tsp ginger, ½ tsp cinnamon. Beat till peaks are strong. Top the hot pancakes with the cream.

BUTTERMILK PANCAKES

Buttermilk pancakes
>2 eggs
>2 2/3 cups buttermilk

½ tsp baking soda

½ tsp salt

4 T sugar

2 tsp baking powder

2 2/3 cups flour

½ cup melted butter

Sift the dry ingredients together in a bowl and set aside. Separate the eggs. Beat the yolks with the buttermilk till fluffy. Beat the egg whites separately till firm peaks form. Add the buttermilk and egg mixture to the dry ingredients and beat well. Fold in the egg whites. Fry the pancakes till golden on each side.

42

CREPES

Crepes
   1 cup cake flour, sifted
   ½ cup powdered sugar
¼ tsp salt
1 cup milk or cream
3 eggs, beaten light and foamy
¼ tsp flavoring, I like almond
Filling:
1 pkg. cream cheese, softened to room temperature
1 jar strawberry topping, usually sold next to ice cream
½ cup sugar

Sift the dry ingredients in the crepe section. Add the milk or cream and beat till smooth. Add the eggs and flavoring. Mix well. Beat the cream cheese and the sugar. Set aside. Fry the crepes on a griddle they should be thin. Spread with the cream cheese mixture, top with the strawberry topping and roll up. Add more strawberry topping on top of the rolled crepe.

43

CHOCOLATE PECAN PANCAKES

Chocolate pecan pancakes
  1 pkg. chocolate pudding mix
  ¼ cup sugar
1 cup flour
1 tsp baking powder
½ cup milk
1 cup pecans, chopped
½ tsp salt
2 eggs
½ cup melted butter

Sift together the dry ingredients. Beat the eggs well. Add the butter, then the milk, beat between. Add the dry mixture. Stir well. Add the nuts. Fry on both sides till done. Top with chocolate sauce and whipped cream.

FUDGE SAUCE

Fudge sauce
    1 ½ cups heavy cream
    2 cups sugar
4 oz. unsweetened baking chocolate
¼ cup butter
1 tsp rum
½ tsp salt
¼ cup instant coffee
Heat cream and sugar to a rolling boil. Stir constantly for 1-2 minutes. Add the chocolate and coffee and stir till melted. Beat over heat till smooth. Remove from heat and add the butter rum and salt. Beat to smooth it out.

45

SOUPS

Soups:

1. KIMMY'S POTATO SOUP
2. BROCCOLI SOUP
3. CHEESEBURGER SOUP
4. CAULIFLOWER SOUP
5. GRANDMA'S CHILI
6. AUTUMN SQUASH SOUP
7. CHICKEN AND WILD RICE SOUP

BEHOLD, I stand at the door and knock: if any man hear my voice, and open the door, I will come into him, and will sup with him, and he with me. Revelation 3:20

KIMMY'S POTATO SOUP

Kimmy's Potato Soup
1 bag of medium sized potatoes
2 small cartons of sour cream
1 stick of butter
1 pkg. shredded Colby Jack cheese
2 pkg bacon bits
Seasoned salt
Garlic powder
Onion powder
Mrs. Dash garlic and herb blend

Peel and chop the potatoes into a large pot. Barely cover them with water, not completely, some potatoes should be sticking out of the water. Boil with a lid on for as long as it takes for the potatoes to be so tender they fall apart when tested with a fork. Drain a tiny bit of the water off the top or cook on low heat to evaporate some. The water should be in 2/3 of the pot. The vitamins that cooked out of the potatoes is in this water, so we use it in the soup. Mash the potatoes into the remaining water. Mash out all the lumps that are large. Add the seasonings to taste. Add 1 stick of butter cut into pieces. Add the sour cream and bacon. Serve warm.

GRANDMA'S BROCCOLI SOUP

Grandma's **Broccoli soup**
2 bags of frozen broccoli florets
1 stick of butter
2 small cartons of sour cream
Mrs. Dash garlic and herb blend
Garlic powder
Onion powder
Seasoned salt
2 pkgs. shredded Colby Jack cheese
2 pkgs. of bacon bits

Place the broccoli in a large pot and cover barely with water, the tops of the broccoli should be above the water. Boil till the broccoli is so tender its falling apart. Drain off a tiny bit of the water, you still need most of it. The vitamins are in the water. Dump the whole pot, broccoli and water into the blender and puree' it into soup. Pour it back into the big pot it cooked in. Add the butter, the seasonings, the sour cream, the cheese and the bacon. Stir well to blend everything well. Taste it and add seasonings if needed. Serve hot.

CHEESEBURGER SOUP

Cheeseburger soup
   2 pkgs ground sirloin, lean
   1 stick butter
1 onion, chopped
1 cup shredded carrots
1 green pepper, chopped
1 tsp dried basil
1 ½ lbs. potatoes, peeled and chopped
3 cups beef broth
¼ cup flour
2 pkg. cubed soft cheese; Colby will work.
1 ½ cups cream
½ tsp salt
1 cup sour cream
Garlic powder
Onion powder
Chili powder

In a large pot brown, the ground sirloin till no pink shows, add the spices. Add the chopped onion, peppers and carrots, stir fry till the onions are tender, add the basil and potatoes. Cook them till the potatoes are starting to brown. Add the beef broth and turn the heat down to a simmer. Simmer covered with a lid so the potatoes can soften up. 10-12 minutes. In a small skillet melt the butter, add the flour and a few spoons of the broth from the stew. Stir and fry for 5 minutes, then dump the flour mixture into the stew. Cook for 3 more minutes, then add the cream and cheese. Continue to cook it for 3 minutes stirring constantly. Add the sour cream mix well. Taste it to see if you need any seasonings. Add more seasoning as needed. Serve hot with garlic toast.

Garlic toast:

Sourdough bread

1 stick butter melted

½ pack of dry ranch powders

3 T garlic powder

Melt the butter and add the ranch powder and garlic, stir really well. Lay the slices of sourdough on a cookie sheet and paint the melted butter mix on the bread, re-mix the butter mixture often because it separates. Toast the bread in the oven on broil till the top is lightly browned.

CAULIFLOWER SOUP

Cauliflower soup
   2 bags frozen cauliflower florets
   1 pkg. shredded Colby jack cheese
2 small containers sour cream
1 stick of butter
Garlic powder
Onion powder
Seasoned salt
2 pkg bacon bits

Place the cauliflower in a large pot, and barely cover it with water, the tops should be above the water. Boil with a lid, till the cauliflower is so tender it is falling apart. Drain a tiny amount of the water off, keep most of it. Pour it all into a blender, cauliflower and the water it cooked in. Puree' it and pour it back into the pot it cooked in. Add the butter, sour cream and seasonings to taste. Add the cheese and bacon. Reheat to hot and serve hot.

WE USE the water it cooked in because the vitamins that cooked out shouldn't be thrown away.

GRANDMA'S CHILI

Grandma's Chili
2 lbs. ground beef
2 large onions
2-3 cans of Kidney beans
Tomato sauce or puree
Celery chopped
Garlic
Onion powder
Chili powder
Cumin, about ¼ tsp
1 cup water
Salt
Pepper

Fry the onions and celery in a few T of olive oil till caramelized. Set aside. Fry the ground beef, chopping it up and seasoning it with a liberal amount of garlic, onion powder and chili powder, when well done, set it aside. In a large stock pot put the fried beef, the fried onions and celery, the kidney beans, the tomato sauce and the water. Set it on medium heat to slow simmer and add seasonings. Taste it and add more as needed. The salt, pepper, chili powder, garlic, etc. is seasoned to taste. Slow simmer for several hours, checking on it often to add water as needed. The flavors of chili "bloom" and merge together as it slow simmers. Chili is more than food, it's a personal taste exploration.

AUTUMN SQUASH SOUP

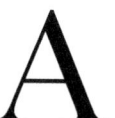utumn Squash soup
3 T butter
8 cups butternut squash cut up
3 carrots cut small
1 onion, chopped
1 T dark brown sugar
1 T maple syrup
½ tsp salt
¼ tsp curry
¼ tsp nutmeg
¼ tsp cinnamon
1/8 tsp cayenne pepper
½ cup pumpkin puree'
1 cup apple juice
3 cups vegetable broth
1 cup coconut milk

Heat butter in a Dutch oven. Add the squash carrots and onion and cook 10 minutes. Add the brown sugar and maple syrup. Add the salt, curry, nutmeg, cinnamon, and cayenne. Cook and stir constantly for 2 minutes. Add the pumpkin, the apple juice and broth, bring to a boil and reduce to simmer. Simmer for 20-25 minutes, till the squash is tender enough to mash easily. Add the coconut milk and stir well. Remove from heat. Puree' the soup in a blender, if you can't fit it all into a blender work in batches. When it's all smoothly puree' pour it into the Dutch oven and heat to desired temperature. Serve with pumpkin seed floaters.

VARIATION: do the same process with sweet potatoes instead of squash.

Chicken and wild rice soup

1 cup wild long grain rice

2 T butter

1 onion, chopped

1 celery stalk, finely sliced

1 carrot, chopped

1 garlic clove, minced

2 T flour

3 cups cream

1 ½ cups chicken broth

2 cups chicken, cooked and chopped

Cook the rice following the package instructions and set aside. Add the chicken to the rice and mix well. Set aside. In a large pot melt the butter and stir fry the onion and celery till tender. Add the garlic and flour and stir a bit more till the flour starts to change color. Add the chicken broth, boil 2 minutes, stirring constantly. Add the cream and turn down the heat to simmer, stir till it begins to thicken. Add the rice and chicken mixture, add any seasonings to taste. Simmer for a few minutes. Serve hot

MEATS

Meats:

1. GRANDMA'S CHICKEN KIEV STYLE WITH SOUR CREAM GRAVY
2. CHICKEN CHILI
3. CHICKEN AND WACKY MAC CASSEROLE
4. POT ROAST
5. GRANDMA'S FAST CHICKEN AND GRAVY FOR BUSY MOMS
6. HAMBURGER STEAKS
7. BEEF BBQ
8. KIMMY'S MEATLOAF
9. KIMMY'S PESTO CHICKEN LASAGNA
10. LASAGNA WITH BEEF
11. BEEF HASH
12. CROCK POT SWISS STEAK
13. KIMMY'S CHICKEN CASSEROLE
14. KIMMY'S FRIED CORNBREAD CAKES WITH ROAST
15. KIMMY'S CHICKEN AND RICE BAKE
16. KIMMY'S CHICKEN HASHBROWN CASSEROLE
17. STEAK IN A SACK
18. KIMMY'S CHICKEN ALFREDO

Pleasant words are as an honeycomb, sweet to the soul, and health to the bones. Proverbs 16:24

GRANDMA'S CHICKEN KIEV STYLE WITH SOUR CREAM GRAVY

Grandma's Chicken Kiev style with Sour Cream Gravy
(This is not diet food, and it isn't low fat either)
Raw Chicken breasts, boneless and skinless
Thinly sliced deli ham
Bacon
Cream of celery soup
1 pint of sour cream
Garlic
Onion powder
Flatten the chicken breasts as flat as possible and top each one with a slice or two of the ham. Fold each breast in ½ long ways, with the ham inside the chicken breast. Wrap each breast with a strip of the raw bacon and lay them side by side in a baking dish. When all the chicken is in the pan season the tops of the chicken with the garlic and onion powder. Cover the dish with aluminum foil and bake at 350F for 3 hours. Take the pan out of the oven and mix the sour cream and the can of soup together in a bowl. Pour the sour cream mixture over the chicken and return to the oven at the same temperature as before for 45 minutes. The bacon drippings in the pan and the soup and sour cream will mix flavors, this is amazing, but not for those trying to eat low fat. For a low-fat version, you can use turkey bacon and fat free sour cream, but you need to add some fluid to the pan for the 3 hours of baking, a little chicken stock should work. Serve hot with mashed potatoes

CHICKEN CHILI

C hicken Chili
    3-4 cups cooked chicken, chopped
    1 large can tomato puree'
2-3 cans dark red kidney beans
Garlic powder
Chili powder
Mrs. Dash garlic and herb blend
½ jar Alfredo sauce

Stir fry the chicken with seasonings to taste, then place it in a large pot on the stove with the tomato puree', the kidney beans and season it to taste while it simmers on low heat for 1-2 hours stirring often. When the flavors seem to blend well and you like the taste, add the Alfredo sauce and simmer for 30 more minutes to blend all flavors. Stir often.

Variation: seasoning varies a lot due to personal preferences. You might try oregano and basil or cumin as spices to try.

CHICKEN AND WACKY MAC CASSEROLE

Chicken and wacky mac casserole
2 cans chunk chicken, the large sizes
1 jar Alfredo sauce
1 bag wacky mac rotini pasta
Garlic
Chili powder
Mrs. Dash
Salt and pepper
1-2 pkg. shredded cheese

Stir fry the chicken in the spices to taste. I use a lot of garlic and a good bit of the chili powder. When it is incorporated well set it aside. Boil the wacky mac but just until it bends, don't overcook it because we will be baking it too, which also softens it. When its just starting to bend, remove it from the heat, drain the water out and add in the chicken. Stir it well to blend. Add the Alfredo sauce and mix well. Pour the whole casserole into a baking dish and top with cheese. Bake at 350 for 40 minutes, or until it is hot and bubbly and the top starts to brown. At this point you can add panko and just crisp the top if you like a crunchy topping. Serve hot.

POT ROAST

P ot roast

    2 medium roasts or 1 if you live alone

    Russet potatoes, 6 or however many you like

Carrots cut into baby carrot size, one bag

1-2 onions, cut in quarters

Garlic powder

Onion powder

Seasoned salt, or other salt

Place the meat in a large Dutch oven with a lid, or a turkey roaster with a lid. Wash the potatoes to get off any dust and rinse the carrots. Add 2-3 cups of water to the pan around the roast. Season the meat and water heavily with the seasonings, less salt than the other two spices. Add the vegetables in snugly around the roast you can also cover the meat if necessary, the steam made from the baking will soften them. Cover the pan and bake in the oven at 350F for 3 hours. If your pan doesn't have a lid use aluminum foil, it works just as well. After the 3 hours its ready to serve.

GRANDMA'S FAST CHICKEN AND GRAVY FOR BUSY MOMS

G randma's fast chicken and gravy for busy Moms
　　6-8 chicken breasts, boned and skinned
　　2 cans cream of celery soup
½ jar of Alfredo sauce
Garlic powder
Onion powder

Lay the chicken breasts in a baking pan side by side. Season the meat with the garlic and onion powder, I use a good bit. In a large bowl, mix the soup and the Alfredo sauce. Pour it over the chicken in the pan. Cover with aluminum foil and bake in the oven at 400F for 3-4 hours till the chicken has no pink inside. Serve with your favorite vegetables, we like it with potatoes.

HAMBURGER STEAKS

Hamburger steaks
    2 packages of lean ground sirloin
    ½ bottle A-1 steak sauce
2 onions, sliced
Garlic powder
Chili powder
Onion powder

Dump the sirloin in a large mixing bowl and add the A-1 sauce. Mix the sauce into the meat by kneading it with your hands or using a large heavy metal spoon to cut the meat and mash the meat, with the sauce until it is well blended. Make hamburger patties with the meat and season each side liberally with garlic, onion and chili powders. Fry on both sides in a skillet with a lid, till its as done as you like. Lower the heat to simmer, add the sliced onions and some water in the pan to simmer till the onions are tender. Serve with your favorite veggies.

BEEF BBQ

Beef BBQ
Pot roast, already baked and shredded
1 large can tomato puree'
2 T molasses
1 T liquid smoke
1 cup coke-a-cola
1 tsp onion powder
3 T garlic powder
3 T chili powder
Salt to taste

Mix all the ingredients in a saucepan on the stove over low heat, except the meat. Slow simmer and taste, add more seasoning if needed. Add brown sugar if it's not sweet enough. Slow cook it while stirring often. Place the meat in a crock pot and pour the sauce over it. Slow cook on low for 2-3 hours.

60

KIMMY'S MEATLOAF

Kimmy's Meatloaf
2 lbs. of ground beef (the leaner the better)
Breadcrumbs, or stovetop stuffing
2 eggs
Garlic and any seasoning you like
1 large onion chopped and fried till caramelized
1 bottle A-1 steak sauce

Mix the eggs, onion, and the breadcrumbs into the meat. Season it with garlic, salt, chili powder, onion powder. Mix the A-1 sauce into the meat and incorporate everything well. Bake at 350F for 3 hours. Serve with mashed potatoes or a favorite vegetable. I top it with aluminum foil and then remove the aluminum foil the last 20 minutes to brown the top.

KIMMY'S PESTO CHICKEN LASAGNA

Kimmy's Pesto Chicken Lasagna
    3 Chicken breasts, boneless and skinless
    1 can tomato puree
½ jar Alfredo sauce
3 T crushed garlic in olive oil
3 T basil, dried
3 T oregano, dried
Juice from 1 lemon
Black walnuts, about 1 cup, finely crushed
1 box lasagna noodles
1 large carton cottage cheese
2 pkg. shredded mozzarella cheese
1 pkg. Colby jack shredded cheese
½ stick butter
Olive oil for sauté' of spices
1 T rosemary
3 T garlic powder

In a saucepan on low heat sauté' the garlic in olive oil, basil, oregano, lemon juice and black walnuts. We want it to smell less herbal and more like spices to cook with about 3 minutes, stirring constantly, be careful not to scorch it. Set it aside. In a baking dish lay the chicken and cover it with the sautéed pesto mix. Add 2 cups of water to the pan, but don't displace the spices on the chicken, try to pour it into the edges. Top the pan with foil and bake on 350F for 3 hours, till no pink is inside the chickens. Take the chicken out and shred it into small pieces, coating it with the spices. Set it aside. Now we get a pot and lightly boil the lasagna noodles just until they are bendy. You don't want them soft; they will soften in the baking. Drain out the water and in the baking pan we used for the chicken we will build the lasagna. Scoop the chicken out into a bowl. In another bowl mix the tomato puree and alfredo sauce. Add the chicken and mix well. Scoop just enough of the chicken and sauce into the baking pan to cover the bottom. Add a layer of lasagna noodles on top. Cover the noodles with cottage cheese and the shredded cheese, be sure to save some cottage and shredded cheese for another layer. Add another layer of chicken then add more noodles and the cheeses. More chicken, hopefully the last of it, and top with the cheeses. Bake in the oven on 350F for an hour. The top should be golden and the sauce bubbly.

LASAGNA WITH BEEF

L asagna, with beef
2 pkgs. of lean ground sirloin
1 large can tomato puree'
4 T Garlic powder
3 T Onion powder
5-6 T chili powder
3 T oregano
2 T dried basil
2 T rosemary
1 box lasagna noodles
½ stick butter
2 large cartons of cottage cheese
2 pkg. shredded mozzarella cheese
2 pkg. shredded Colby Jack cheese
2 pkg. shredded taco cheese

Stir fry the ground meat in a skillet and season it heavily with the garlic, onion and chili powder. When no pink shows, add the oregano, basil and rosemary. Add the tomato sauce and turn down the heat to a simmer. Stir often and simmer around 20 minutes. Set aside. Boil the lasagna noodles till they just start to bend well, don't overcook, we will be baking them, and they soften the rest of the way in the baking pan. Now we add the butter to the noodles to keep them from sticking together. In a large baking pan layer, the lasagna this way:

Meat sauce on the bottom, a layer of noodles, cottage cheese in a thin layer, lots of shredded cheese, now more meat, then the noodles then the cheeses, in layers, the last layer is meat and cheese only. Cover with a lid or parchment paper then aluminum foil and bake at 350F for an hour. Serve hot. Preferably with garlic bread.

Warning: Do not ever store any food with a tomato sauce in aluminum, it will eat flakes loose and the flakes will be in your food!! We transfer any tomato-based food to a plastic container for storage. And don't cover tomato-based foods with only aluminum foil, the same thing happens. Always have a barrier like wax paper or parchment paper over the tomato-based food then aluminum can be used over the paper.

BEEF HASH

Beef Hash
2 lb. ground beef
Several Irish potatoes, peeled and chopped
1 large onion
1 green pepper
Garlic
Onion powder
Chili powder
1T Any cooking oil for frying, we like olive oil

Fry the onion and green pepper in oil till well caramelized, add the beef and season it well with the garlic, onion powder and chili powder. Continue frying till the beef is well done, add the chopped potatoes and continue to cook till the potatoes soften and form brown crusty edges. If you allow the potatoes to brown before stirring them up, it will form nice nonstick edges, some will stick, just because potatoes are starchy.

CROCK POT SWISS STEAK

Crock pot Swiss steak
4 Chopped steaks
1 green tomato (an unripe one), peeled and chopped
Flour for dredging
Beef bullion
Beef stock
1 stick butter
Seasoned salt
Pepper

Dredge the steaks in flour, season with salt and pepper, and start browning them in the butter in a skillet. When both sides are seared, transfer the meat to a crock pot. Add some flour to the pan drippings and continue stirring to brown the flour into a rue. Add beef bouillon and a tiny bit of the beef broth, continue to stir, forming a gravy. When the gravy is thick add it to the crockpot. Add the green tomato and the remaining beef stock. Stir and simmer for 5-6 hours on low heat. Check it often to be sure it's not drying out. When the steak is tender, and the sauce thick it is done.

KIMMY'S CHICKEN CASSEROLE

K immy's Chicken Casserole
  2 pkg. chicken tenders, chopped
  2 cups brown rice, cooked
½ jar Alfredo sauce
4 slices bacon
1 can cream of celery soup
½ cup sour cream
3 potatoes, peeled and chopped
1 pkg. grated cheese

Fry the bacon, and set it aside, toss in the potatoes and fry them in the bacon grease. When the potatoes are done spoon them out of the pan, onto the plate with the bacon. Fry the chicken till no pink shows, in the same skillet add butter as needed. When the chicken is done, all sides browned, set it aside. In a large bowl put the rice, the chicken the bacon, broken up into pieces, the Alfredo, the celery soup, the sour cream and mix everything well. In a large baking pan pour the chicken mixture and add the potatoes push the potatoes into the mixture till they are just covered. Top the casserole with the shredded cheese and bake at 350F till hot and bubbly.

KIMMY'S FRIED CORNBREAD CAKES WITH ROAST

K immy's Fried Cornbread cakes with roast

2 cups cornmeal

½ cup butter, melted

1 egg

Buttermilk

Cooked and shredded roast beef

½ cup Alfredo sauce

1 cup shredded cheese

Mix all the ingredients, except the beef, and make it soupy by adding more milk as needed to make a runny pancake consistency. Add the beef and mix well. Fry like pancakes, let each side turn golden brown before flipping to the uncooked side. I fry in butter, but you can use cooking oil or bacon grease.

KIMMY'S CHICKEN AND RICE BAKE

K immy's Chicken and Rice bake
2 cans chunk chicken, well chopped
2 cups brown rice, cooked following the package instructions
1 can cream of chicken soup
½ jar Alfredo sauce
1 pkg. shredded cheese
Garlic
Dash
Panko breadcrumbs
Sliced almonds, sauté' in butter till golden

Mix the chicken, rice, seasoning, soup and Alfredo sauce. Pour into a 9X13 baking pan and top with cheese. Bake at 350F till hot and bubbly. Top with the panko mixed with the almonds, and heat till the top is nicely crisp. Remove from the oven and serve.

KIMMY'S CHICKEN HASH-BROWN CASSEROLE

Kimmy's Chicken hash-brown casserole
2 cans chunk chicken, well chopped
2 bags French fried onions
1 can cream of chicken soup
½ jar Alfredo sauce
1 large bag sliced almonds
1 small bag frozen hash-brown potatoes
1 stick butter
Garlic, salt and dash to taste

Fry the hash-browns in the butter till nicely browned. Mix the hash-browns, the soup, Alfredo and the chicken together in a large bowl. Season to taste. Pour into a 9X13 baking pan and bake at 350F till hot. Top with the fried onions and almonds, bake till the top browns nicely, about 3 minutes. Serve hot.

STEAK IN A SACK

S teak in a sack
  1 pkg. ground sirloin, lean
  1 pkg. pita bread
1 onion, chopped
1 green pepper, chopped
Garlic powder, chili powder, onion powder, season to taste
Butter to fry the sandwiches
Fry the beef till no pink shows, toss in the onion and pepper and cook till tender. Add the spices to taste. Cut open the pita bread by ½ to make 2 pockets. Stuff the pita pockets with the meat mixture. Fry the pita pocket sandwiches on both sides in butter till crisp and golden. Serve hot.

KIMMY'S CHICKEN ALFREDO

K immy's Chicken Alfredo
6 chicken breasts, boned and skinned
1 jar Alfredo sauce.

½ carton sour cream

2 T garlic powder

2 T dry ranch powder, in the salad dressing aisle at the grocery store

6 slices of raw bacon

Lay the chicken breasts in a large baking pan and top with the bacon. In a large bowl mix the Alfredo sauce, the sour cream, the garlic and ranch. Mix till well combined. Pour the sauce over the chicken and top the pan with aluminum foil. Bake at 350F for 3 hours or till done.

CHICKEN BACON STEW

Chicken Bacon stew
    6 chicken breasts, cooked and chopped
    8 slices of bacon
1 jar Alfredo sauce
1 can cream of celery soup
1 small carton sour cream
1 small can chicken broth
Garlic to taste
Onion powder to taste

Fry the bacon, save the grease to fry the chicken till nice and brown on all sides, add the garlic and continue to fry the to blend the flavors. Dump it all into a big pot, including any bacon grease in the pan. In a large bowl mix the Alfredo, celery soup and sour cream. Add to the pot add the chicken broth and mix everything well. Put on the simmer setting of low heat. Add garlic and onion powder to taste. Let simmer for an hour, stirring often. You can use a crock pot if you want an easier low stir option. Serve with garlic bread.

HOPE AND FAITH'S PESTO CHICKEN

Hope and Faith's Pesto Chicken
>   5 Chicken breasts, boneless and skinless
>   3 T crushed garlic in olive oil

1 cup basil, dried

1/3 cup oregano, dried

Juice from 1 lemon

Black walnuts, about 1 cup, finely crushed

Olive oil for sauté' of spices

1/4 cup garlic powder

1/3 cup parmesan cheese, powdered kind

Soak the herbs in the saucepan for 5 minutes in 1/3 cup water. In the saucepan on low heat sauté' the garlic in olive oil, basil, oregano, lemon juice, and black walnuts. We want it to smell less herbal and more like spices to cook with about 3 minutes, stirring constantly, be careful not to scorch it. Add 1/3 cup parmesan cheese, powder right before removing from heat. Set it aside. In a baking dish lay the chicken and cover it with the sautéed pesto mix. Add 2 cups of water to the pan, but don't displace the spices on the chicken, try to pour it into the edges. Top the pan with foil and bake on 350F for 4 hours, till no pink is inside the chickens. Serve hot with a favorite veggie.

GRILLED FLOUNDER

Grilled Flounder
    6 Frozen Flounder filets
    Worcestershire sauce
1 stick of butter, melted
Dry ranch powder (found in the salad dressing aisle)
Garlic powder

Lay the frozen filets on a baking sheet. The melted butter will be in a measuring cup you can pour from. Mix a bit of the ranch powder in the butter to season it. Don't use a whole packet its very strong just mix maybe 1/8 of the packet into the butter. Lightly coat the fish fillets with the butter mixture and sprinkle some Worcestershire sauce on each filet. Broil till the fish turns white, and firm to the touch on both sides. Season each side the same way as you broil. Serve with more butter sauce poured over the fish. Be sure to mix the butter sauce often because it separates.

SHRIMP SCAMPI HACK

Shrimp scampi hack
     15 shrimp deveined and cleaned
     3 T garlic powder
1/8 package dry ranch powder (the type used to make ranch dressing)
1 stick butter, melted
2 cloves garlic minced
Olive oil

Lay the shrimp in a ceramic or glass baking dish, sprinkle with garlic powder. In a measuring cup mix the dry ranch, the garlic cloves, the melted butter and a few tablespoons of olive oil, pour it over the shrimp. Cook under the broiler, rotating often be sure to baste it with the butter mixture often. When the shrimp is done, its pink and white and firm. Remove from the heat and serve with rice, pour the remaining sauce from the baking pan over the shrimp and the rice.

KIMMY'S TROPICAL CHICKEN SALAD

Kimmy's tropical chicken salad
3 large cans of chunk chicken
Green grapes cut into quarters, about 4 cups worth
1 pkg shredded coconut
2 cups pecans, chopped
2 individual size cherry flavored Greek yogurts

Mix all the ingredients well and serve on toasted croissants or your favorite bread.

Variation: you can do the same thing with any left-over chicken breast.

SAUSAGE BALLS

S ausage Balls
    1 pkg sausage
    1 pkg. shredded cheese
2 cups bisquick baking mix
1/8 package dry ranch powders

Put the bisquick in a large bowl. Add the dry ranch powders and mix well. Add the cheese. Stir fry the sausage till no pink appears. Dump the fried sausage including any grease it made into the bisquick and mix well to form a dough. Make balls from the dough and bake on a cookie sheet in the oven at 350F for a few minutes till the balls look golden brown. Serve hot.

Variation: for those who cannot have sausage, use chunk chicken and fry it in melted butter. Season the chicken with garlic powder and onion powder. Use a bit more melted butter as needed if the dough is too dry.

BEEF STROGANOFF

Beef Stroganoff
   2 lbs. sirloin steaks sliced then cubed
   2 onions, sliced thin
1 clove garlic, minced. (you can buy it already minced in olive oil)
½ cup butter
1 can beef broth
1 tsp Worcestershire sauce
1/8 pkg. dry ranch powders
1 carton sour cream
3 cups cooked noodles, curly ones
3 T flour

Fry the meat and onion in the butter till brown. Add ½ the beef broth and simmer 15 minutes. Mix the flour into the other ½ of the beef broth and add it. Mix in the sour cream, the Worcestershire sauce, the ranch powders and let simmer for 12-15 minutes for the sauce to thicken up. Serve hot over the noodles.

HOPE'S TUNA PATTIES

Hope's Tuna Patties
These are like the salmon patties but with tuna. They are eggless for those with sensitivity to eggs.

2 large cans of tuna (12 oz.)

½ jar Alfredo sauce

2 cups shredded cheese, Colby is good

2 T garlic powder

2 T Mrs. Dash garlic blend

1 T chili powder

2 cups crushed potato chips

Mix all the ingredients together in a large bowl, it needs to be sticky enough to form patties like hamburger patties but much thinner. Fry in olive oil, till both sides are golden brown and crispy. We wait to flip them till the underside is really crispy to keep them from falling apart. The soft shredded cheese and Alfredo help to act as tasty glue, but patience is required for success.

SALMON PATTIES

Salmon Patties
2-3 cans of salmon, you can buy it already cleaned or go thru it and pick out the bones and skin.
½ jar Alfredo sauce
2 cups shredded Colby cheese or mozzarella
2 T garlic powder
2 T Mrs. Dash, garlic blend
2 T chili powder, trust me its delicious
2 cups crushed potato chips
Mix all the ingredients together and form patties, like hamburger patties but thinner. Fry the patties in olive oil till golden and crispy on both sides. Wait to flip the patty till the underside is crispy to keep it intact. Serve hot with veggies.

VEGGIES

Veggies:

1. GREEN BEAN CASSEROLE
2. THOSE MASHED POTATOES WITH ALMONDS
3. CORN CASSEROLE
4. FRIED POTATOES
5. FRIED OKRA
6. HOPE'S ORANGE CRANBERRY BUTTERNUT SQUASH
7. KIMMY'S BACON FRIED RICE
8. KIMMY'S CREAM SPINACH BAKE
9. FRIED GREEN TOMATOES
10. FAITH'S PEPPERS AND ONIONS ON THE GRILL
11. OLD TIMEY PINTO BEANS
12. CINNAMON CARROTS
13. CHILI SPICE GREEEN BEANS

IF YE BE willing and obedient, ye shall eat the good of the land. Isaiah 1:19

GREEN BEAN CASSEROLE

Green Bean Casserole
  2 bags frozen French style green beans
  2 cans of cream of celery soup
1 pkg bacon bits
French fried onions
Sliced almonds
Garlic
Onion powder
Seasoned salt

In a large bowl mix the green beans, the soup, the bacon and the seasonings. Pour all of it into a baking pan and bake at 350F for 40 minutes. Add the fried onions and sliced almonds on top and bake till it browns. Serve hot

THOSE MASHED POTATOES WITH ALMONDS

Those Mashed Potatoes with Almonds
I ½ bag russet potatoes
2 sticks of butter
I large carton sour cream
I small cream cheese, softened
I pkg. grated Colby jack cheese
Garlic, seasoned salt and onion powder to taste
I lg pkg 12oz sliced almonds

Scrub and peel the potatoes and cut them into cubes, put them in a large pot and cover with water. Cook on Medium till the potatoes are tender enough to fall apart, this keeps the mashed potatoes from being lumpy. When soft, pull the potatoes off the heat and drain the water off. Dump the potatoes into a kitchen aid or similar mixer, add one stick of butter and start mixing on medium then switch to high speed. When smooth, stop the mixer and add the sour cream and seasonings. Add the cheese, mix well. Sauté' the almonds in a skillet with the remaining stick of butter and when they are a lovely brown, put them into the mixer and mix again. Add the cream cheese. Mix well. Taste it to see if it needs more seasoning. Serve warm

CORN CASSEROLE

Corn casserole
2 cups fresh or frozen corn
2 T sugar
Dash of pepper
1 cup evaporated milk
1 tsp salt
4 eggs
2 T butter

Beat the eggs just a bit, and add the corn, set aside. Combine the sugar, salt, pepper and milk, and add to the corn mixture. Beat smooth and pour into a greased baking pan. Drizzle butter over the top and bake at 350F for one hour till firm.

FRIED POTATOES, SOUTHERN STYLE

Fried Potatoes
      4-5 potatoes
      Bacon, around 5 pieces
1 large onion, chopped
1 large green pepper, chopped
Garlic
Salt and pepper
Chili powder

Start frying the bacon, when it is done enough to suit you, put it on a plate and set aside, but leave the bacon grease in the pan, and add the onions and peppers to start them, after they soften a bit add the potatoes and the spices, and stir fry till the potatoes are browned, tender and crispy on the outside, add the bacon back to the pan, breaking it up as you add it. Keep stirring and cooking on low, till all the ingredients are well mixed and flavors incorporated. Serve hot, top with cheese if you like.

FRIED OKRA

Fried Okra
A bag full of tender young okra, use your fingernail when buying to be sure each one is soft, short pieces are better than older long ones that may be tough.

2 cups cornmeal to dredge

Seasoned salt

Garlic

Olive oil for frying

Slice the okra into slices. Dredge in the corn meal, and add to the skillet with the olive oil to fry to a dark crispy brown. Salt with the seasoned salt while frying. You want the okra to be crispy tap it with a metal spoon to test it. Okra flavor changes the more it cooks. Taste a dark piece and a lighter piece to test the difference. When its crispy drain it on paper towels in a baking pan, in an oven set to 250F. serve hot

HOPE'S ORANGE CRANBERRY BUTTERNUT SQUASH

Hope's Orange cranberry Butternut Squash
2-4 pkg frozen butternut squash
1 pkg frozen cranberries
½ tsp grated orange rind
¼ cup orange juice
¼ cup butter
¼ cup dark brown sugar, packed
½ tsp salt
1 tsp cinnamon
½ tsp ginger
¼ tsp nutmeg

Put the frozen squash in a saucepan, cover and cook on medium heat. About 15 minutes. Check it for any hard spots and remove those they won't soften later. Stir in all the remaining ingredients. Pour it into a baking dish and bake at 350F for 45 minutes. Make a crumb topping to go on top.

Crumb topping:
2 cups rolled oats
1 cup dark brown sugar
1 stick melted butter
1 cup pecans, chopped

Mix all the ingredients into a crumbly mix and top the squash, brown it a bit in the oven to make it crisp

KIMMY'S BACON FRIED RICE

K immy's Bacon Fried Rice
6 bacon slices
1 large onion, chopped
1 large green pepper, chopped
Quick rice, like the rice-a-Roni type
2 T soy sauce
2 T sesame oil
Sliced almonds, about ½ a large bag
Garlic

Start frying the bacon, when done enough to suit, set it on a plate and put it aside, but leave the grease in the pan. Add the onions and green pepper and stir fry them till they are tender. Add the rice and brown it a bit, add the almonds and the soy sauce and the sesame oil, and break up the bacon and add it, add the water amount the quick rice package calls for and simmer till the water is absorbed by the rice.

KIMMY'S CREAM SPINACH BAKE

K immy's Cream Spinach bake
2 pkgs. frozen spinach
1 cup sour cream
1 small pkg. cream cheese, at room temperature for 2 hours
1 small bag grated cheese, Colby jack will work
½ pkg. dry onion soup mix
Garlic
2 tsp lemon juice
Panko breadcrumbs

Cook the spinach briefly in olive oil and garlic, drain if it produces a lot of fluid, don't overcook, we will be baking it too. Mix the sour cream and cream cheese till smooth. Mix in the soup mix and your spinach, blend well. Pour into a well buttered baking dish and bake at 350F for 25 minutes. Top with the panko breadcrumbs and cheese bake till the top is golden brown and the spinach bubbly. Serve hot

FRIED GREEN TOMATOES

F ried Green tomatoes
4 green tomatoes, sliced, these are not a green variety they are unripe red tomatoes, the unripe tomatoes are wonderful fried

2 cups cornmeal for dredging

Seasoned salt

Garlic

Olive oil for frying

Wet the sliced green tomatoes and dredge them in the cornmeal. Salt both sides and drop them in the skillet in the olive oil to fry. Wait to flip them till the bottom is nice and golden brown. When both sides are golden lay them on paper towels in a baking pan to stay warm in an oven set to 250F. serve hot

FAITH'S PEPPERS AND ONIONS ON THE GRILL

Faith's Peppers and Onions on the grill
    3 large peppers
    2 large onions
1 bottle Italian salad dressing

Chop the onions and peppers into whatever size you want. Lay them on aluminum foil that has a large margin around the veggies. Fold up the sides of the foil to form a tent enclosing the veggies on all sides, leave the top open to pour in some Italian dressing. Seal the top edges. Lay it on a grill after the burgers are done and let the heat from the grill cook them and steam them done.

OLD TIMEY PINTO BEANS

Old timey pinto beans
1 pkg. dry pinto beans
3-4 large chunks of ham
1 stick of butter
1 T baking soda

Place the beans in a pot and cover them with water to soak overnight. Add the baking soda, put them on the stove to soak. The next day, drain the water off, and look thru the beans for any pebbles, sometimes the company packaging beans gets pebbles in them. When the beans look clean, rinse them, and cover them with fresh water, add the stick of butter and the ham. Set them on the stove at low heat to simmer for a few hours. Check them often to be sure they don't boil dry. Add water as needed and continue to simmer until they are tender. Taste them often to see if they are tender enough. When they are tender you can add salt. We don't add salt during the simmer because it can stop them from becoming tender. Add whatever seasonings you normally use; I use a lot of garlic in mine. Serve hot with cornbread.

CINNAMON CARROTS

Cinnamon carrots
1 pkg frozen carrot slices
3 T butter
1 T cinnamon
1/8 cup honey

Stir fry the carrots almost done in the butter. Add the cinnamon and honey and continue to cook on low heat till tender. This is popular with the kids.

KIMMY'S CHILI SPICE GREEN BEANS

Kimmy's Chili spice green beans
1-2 pkg. frozen green beans
3 T olive oil
2 T garlic powder
2 T Mrs. Dash garlic blend
3 T chili powder

Stir fry the green beans in the olive oil and spices till tender enough to suit. This is a great side dish for Mexican or Italian style foods.

DESSERTS

D esserts:

1. RUM BUTTER CAKE
2. HUMMINGBIRD CAKE
3. ORANGE PECAN PIE
4. ORANGE MARMALADE CAKE
5. CHOCOLATE MINT MOUSSE PIE
6. COCOA FUDGE
7. DARK CHOCOLATE COCOA CAKE
8. MICROWAVE EASY NO FAIL DIVINITY FUDGE
9. PINEAPPLE MARSHMALLOW PIE
10. HERSHEY'S CHOCOLATE ALMOND BAR PIE
11. ORANGE MARSHMALLOW PIE IN A GINGER CRUST
12. FLUFFY FIVE-MINUTE FROSTING
13. CREAM CHEESE FUDGE
14. BUTTERSCOTCH BOILED FROSTING
15. MARSHMALLOW FROSTING
16. PEANUT BUTTER FROSTING
17. OLD TIMEY CORNSTARCH PUDDING
18. MERINGUE
19. CHIFFON LAYER CAKE

20. CHOCOLATE CHIFFON CAKE
21. LEMON CRUMBLY CRUNCH
22. GRANDMA'S APPLE CAKE
23. KIMMY'S ORANGE SUGAR COOKIES
24. PECAN PIE WITH CHOCOLATE
25. BROWNIE PIE
26. GRANDMA'S BLACK WALNUT CAKE
27. ORANGE NUT BREAD
28. ORANGE CREAM CHEESE FROSTING
29. LEMONADE PIE
30. OLD TIMEY APPLE PIE
31. CRÈME DE MENTHE MARSHMALLOW PIE
32. KEY LIME PIE
33. PECAN CRUST SWEET POTATO PIE
34. ORANGE SLICE CAKE
35. NO BAKE CHERRY CHEESE PIE
36. KIMMY'S ALMOND COOKIES
37. KIMMY'S CHRISTMAS BROWNIES
38. KIMMY'S CHOCOLATE AND LACE COOKIES
39. KARO PECAN PIE
40. SUPER EASY FROZEN MINT PIE
41. KIMMY'S CHOCOLATE MINT CHEESECAKE (FOR DIABETICS)
42. KIMMY'S EASY CHOCOLATE CHIP CHEESECAKE
43. KIMMY'S PUMPKIN PIE
44. HOPE'S PUMPKIN PIE VARIATION FOR DIABETICS
45. APPLE PIE
46. KIMMY'S CHOCOLATE COCONUT ALMOND CHEESECAKE
47. FUDGE FILLED CHEESECAKE
48. EASY FUDGE
49. DOUBLE CHOCOLATE AND BUTTERSCOTCH CHIP COOKIES
50. PECAN DATE CAKE
51. CHOCOLATE ORANGE GANACHE FROSTING
52. CHOCOLATE TRUFFLE CAKE (FLOURLESS CHOCOLATE CAKE)
53. TRIPLE LAYER CHEESECAKE

54. MOCHA FUDGE CAKE
55. ESPRESSO CHOCOLATE CHEESECAKE
56. HERSHEY'S KISSES COOKIES
57. HOT WATER PIE CRUST
58. GREEN TOMATO PIE
59. CANDIED APPLE PIE
60. STRAWBERRY RHUBARB PIE
61. FRIED APPLE PIES
62. CINNAMON BAKED APPLES
63. COCONUT PIE SHELL
64. TOASTED COCONUT PIE
65. COCONUT PIE OLD FASHIONED VERSION
66. CHOCOLATE COCONUT PIE
67. GINGER SNAPS
68. COFFEE FUDGE
69. PEPPERMINT DIVINITY
70. PECAN PRALINE CHEESECAKE
71. SOUR CREAM FUDGE
72. EASY ALMOND COOKIES
73. NUT CRISPS
74. OLD SOUTHERN GINGERBREAD
75. SOUR CREAM LEMON CAKE
76. CANDIED ORANGE PEEL
77. MINTED CHRISTMAS NUTS
78. CANDIED NUTS

BUTTER AND HONEY shall he eat, that he may know to refuse the evil, and choose the good. Isaiah 7:15

MY SON, eat thou honey, because it is good; and the honeycomb, which is sweet to thy taste: so shall the knowledge of wisdom be unto thy soul: when thou hast found it, then there shall be a reward, and thy expectation shall not be cut off. Proverbs 24:13-14

RUM BUTTER CAKE

Rum Butter Cake
2 sticks of butter
½ cup butter flavored Crisco
3 cups dark brown sugar
5 eggs, well beaten
3 cups flour
½ tsp baking powder
1 cup buttermilk
5 T rum
4 tsp butter flavoring

Cream the butter, shortening, and sugar till fluffy. Add the eggs, which have been beaten to a lemon color. Combine the flour and baking powder and add to the creamed mixture alternating with the buttermilk. Stir in the flavoring and rum. Spoon the mixture into a greased and floured tube pan and bake at 350F for 1 ½ hours or until a toothpick inserted comes out clean. Cool in the pan 10 minutes them turn it out onto a plate. Top with rum butter or caramel icing.

Rum butter frosting:

1 stick butter, 4 cups powdered sugar, 3 tsp rum, ¼ cup bailey's Irish cream. Melt and brown the margarine in a saucepan on low heat. Add the powdered sugar gradually adding cream as needed. Beat in the rum and beat till fluffy. Spread on cake when fluffy and chill the cake till time to serve.

Caramel Rum icing:

1 can sweetened condensed milk, rum. Open the can and put the sweetened condensed milk in a microwave safe bowl. Heat it in the microwave at 2 minutes at a time, stirring in between until the milk starts to change to caramel. It will look like the soft caramel in the O'Charley's caramel pie. When it's a nice spreadable caramel, beat in the rum 1 tsp at a time, and taste it till it suits you. Pour it on the cooled cake.

HUMMINGBIRD CAKE

Hummingbird cake
   3 cups flour
   2 cups sugar
1 tsp baking soda
1 tsp salt
1 tsp cinnamon
3 eggs, beaten
1 cup butter, melted
1 ½ tsp vanilla
1 tsp butter flavoring
1 can crushed pineapple, don't drain it
1 cup pecans, chopped
1 jar maraschino cherries, drained and chopped

Combine flour, sugar, soda, salt and cinnamon in a large mixing bowl. Add the eggs and butter, stir till dry ingredients are moist. Do not beat. Stir in the vanilla, butter flavoring and pineapple. Fold in the nuts and cherries. Spoon the batter into a greased and floured cake pan and bake at 350F for 25-30 minutes or until a toothpick inserted comes out clean. Cool in the pan 10 minutes. Turn gently onto a rack or cake tray to cool. Frost with hummingbird frosting and top with chopped pecans.

Hummingbird frosting: 1 pkg cream cheese softened to room temperature,

½ cup butter softened, 1 pkg powdered sugar, sifted, and 1 tsp vanilla flavoring and 1 tsp almond flavoring. Combine the butter and cream cheese and beat smooth. Add powdered sugar and flavorings, beat again till light and fluffy. Frost the cooled cake. Top with chopped pecans

ORANGE PECAN PIE

Orange Pecan pie
3 eggs, separated
1 2/3 cups condensed milk plus enough orange juice to make 2 ¼ cups fluid
Zest of 1 orange rind
½ cup sugar
Pinch of salt
¼ cup sugar
1/3 cup pecans, chopped
1 unbaked pie shell

Beat egg yolks. Add milk with the orange juice, orange zest, and ½ cup sugar. Blend well. Add salt to egg whites, beat till stiff. Add the ½ cup sugar gradually to the egg whites. Fold the egg whites into the milk and egg mixture. Pour into the pie crust. Sprinkle with the chopped pecans. Bake in a hot oven 425F for 10 minutes, then reduce heat to 300F. Bake for 30 minutes longer.

ORANGE MARMALADE CAKE

O range Marmalade cake
Sift together in a large bowl:
2 ¼ cups cake flour
3 tsp double action baking powder (4 tsp single action if you don't have double)
1 cup sugar
½ tsp salt
Add:
½ cup soft butter
¾ cup milk
Beat on low speed for 2 minutes.
Add:
2 eggs
1 T lemon juice
½ cup orange marmalade

Beat 1 minute. Pour into 2 round greased and floured cake pans. Bake at 350F for 25 minutes, or till a toothpick inserted comes out clean. Cool and top with the icing below.

Icing: cream 4 T soft butter with 3 cups powdered sugar. Add ¼ cup lemon juice and beat to a spreading consistency. Frost the layers. Decorate the center of the top with ¼ cup orange marmalade thinned just a bit with water, not much, just enough to make it easy to handle.

CHOCOLATE MINT MOUSSE PIE

Chocolate Mint mousse pie
1 envelope unflavored gelatin
2 T cold water
¼ cup boiling water
1 cup sugar
½ cup Hershey's cocoa
2 cups cold whipping cream (1 pint)
2 tsp mint flavoring
1 pkg Andes mints, chopped
1 chocolate cookie crust
1 bar semi sweet baking chocolate

Sprinkle the gelatin over the cold water in a bowl, let stand 2 minutes to soften. Add the boiling water, stir until the gelatin is completely dissolved and the mixture is clear. Allow to cool slightly. Mix the sugar and cocoa in a large bowl, add the whipping cream and 1 tsp of the mint flavoring. Beat on medium speed till stiff. Pour in the gelatin mixture, beat to blend well. Spoon the mixture into the crust. Chill. In a double boiler melt the baking chocolate, and the remaining 1 tsp of mint flavoring. Add sugar till sweet enough to suit you. Drizzle the chocolate over the chilled pie and put it back into the fridge to chill.

COCOA FUDGE

C ocoa fudge
    2/3 cup Hershey's cocoa
    3 cups dark brown sugar
1 stick butter
1 cup cream
1 tsp rum

Combine the cocoa, sugar, salt and cream in a heavy saucepan. Bring to a boil, stirring constantly. Cook until it reaches the soft ball stage 234-240F on a candy thermometer. Remove from heat and stir in the butter to melt it. Add the rum. Pour into a buttered pan and chill.

DARK CHOCOLATE COCOA CAKE

D ark Chocolate cocoa cake
    2 cups sugar
    1 ¾ cups flour
¾ cups special dark Hershey's cocoa
1 ½ tsp baking powder
1 ½ tsp baking soda
½ tsp salt
2 eggs
1 cup cream
1 stick butter, melted
2 tsp rum
½ cup instant coffee
1 cup boiling water

Preheat the oven to 350F. Grease and flour the baking pan. Sift together the sugar, flour, cocoa, baking powder, baking soda, and salt in a large bowl. Add the eggs, cream, butter and rum. Mix on medium speed with a mixer for 2 minutes. Add the coffee and boiling water, mix well and pour into the baking pan. Bake at 350F for 30-35 minutes or until a toothpick inserted in the center comes out clean. Cool 10 minutes in the pan, remove to cool all the way on a wire rack.

Dark chocolate frosting:

1 stick butter, 2/3 cup special dark Hershey's cocoa, 3 cups powdered sugar, 1/3 cup heavy cream, 1 tsp rum.

Melt the butter. Stir in the cocoa, alternating with the sugar, and cream. Beat till fluffy and spreading consistency. Stir in the rum.

MICROWAVE EASY NO FAIL DIVINITY FUDGE

Microwave easy no fail divinity fudge
4 cups of sugar
1 cup light corn syrup
¾ cup water
Dash of salt
3 egg whites
1 tsp vanilla
Pecans, chopped

In a 2-quart glass microwave safe casserole dish mix the first 4 ingredients. Cook in the microwave 19 minutes, stopping every 5 minutes to stir. Candy thermometer should read 260F when done. While the syrup cooks in the microwave, beat the egg whites stiff. Gradually pour the hot syrup over the egg whites while beating, till thick and the candy loses its gloss. This may take up to 12 minutes. Add the vanilla and nuts, mix well. Drop by teaspoons onto waxed paper.

PINEAPPLE MARSHMALLOW PIE

Pineapple Marshmallow pie
Graham cracker crust
32 large marshmallows, or 3 cups mini marshmallows
1 can crushed pineapple, don't drain
1 T lemon juice
1 ½ cups heavy whipping cream beaten stiff

Combine the marshmallows, pineapple and lemon juice in a 1 quart microwave safe dish. Cook in the microwave for 2 ½ minutes, stir often till the marshmallows are blended. Chill just a bit to partially set. Fold the pineapple mixture into the beaten whipped topping, pour it into the pie crust and chill for 4 hours. You can garnish the top with toasted crumbled almonds to make it pretty.

HERSHEY'S CHOCOLATE ALMOND BAR PIE

Hershey's chocolate almond bar pie
1 chocolate cookie crust
6 Hershey's chocolate almond bars, broken into pieces
15 large marshmallows
½ cup cream
1 cup heavy whipping cream, whipped stiff

In a double boiler combine the chocolate bar pieces, the marshmallows and the milk. Cook 2 minutes stirring constantly. We want the marshmallows melted. If you need longer, cook till they melt. Remove from the heat and mix till smooth. Cool the mixture. Gently fold in the whipped cream into the cooled chocolate. Pour into the crust and chill for 4 hours.

ORANGE MARSHMALLOW PIE IN A GINGER CRUST

Orange Marshmallow pie in a ginger crust

1 1/3 cup gingersnaps, crushed into crumbs

1 stick butter

Pulse the above ingredients in a food processor and mash into the pie pan to form a crust.

32 large marshmallows, or 3 cups mini marshmallows

1 T grated orange zest

¾ cup orange juice

2 T lemon juice

1 ½ cups whipping cream, beaten stiff

Cool the pie shell while making the filling. Combine the marshmallows, orange peel, and juices in a double boiler. Cook on low heat till the marshmallows are melted and incorporated well. Chill till partially set. Fold marshmallows into the whipped cream, pour it into the ginger crust and chill for 4 hours.

FLUFFY FIVE-MINUTE FROSTING

Fluffy five-minute frosting
2 egg whites, unbeaten
1 ½ cups sugar
1/8 tsp salt
¼ tsp cream of tartar
½ cup cold water
1 T light corn syrup
1 tsp vanilla

Place all ingredients except the vanilla in a double boiler, over boiling water. Using an electric mixer, beat at very low speed until ingredients are mixed well, then raise the speed to high, 4-5 minutes. Mixture needs to form a peak when the beater is lifted. Remove the pan from water, add the vanilla and mix till incorporated. Spread on cake.

CREAM CHEESE FUDGE

Cream cheese fudge
    1 3 oz. pkg cream cheese, softened to room temperature
    2 cups powdered sugar
2 1-oz. squares unsweetened baking chocolate, melted
¼ tsp vanilla or rum if you want rum fudge
Dash of salt
½ cup pecans, chopped small
Place the cheese in a mixing bowl and beat it into creamy texture, you want it soft and smooth. Slowly add and blend in the sugar, a small amount at a time. Add the melted chocolate, mix well. Add the vanilla or rum, salt and the pecans. Mix till well blended. Grease a small square baking pan and put the fudge in it pressing it into the bottom. Chill till set. Cut into squares before letting the kids get ahold of it. If you have a big family, you may want to double the recipe and use a larger pan.

BUTTERSCOTCH BOILED FROSTING

Butterscotch boiled frosting
  2 egg whites
  ½ cup Karo syrup
½ cup dark brown sugar
½ tsp salt
1 tsp vanilla

Combine egg whites, Karo, brown sugar and salt in the top of a double boiler. Place the top over rapidly boiling water and cook, stirring constantly with a rotary beater for 7 minutes till the frosting will stand in peaks. Remove from heat. Add flavoring and beat it in well.

MARSHMALLOW FROSTING

Marshmallow frosting
2 egg whites
¾ cup Karo syrup
¼ cup sugar
1/8 tsp salt
1 ¼ tsp vanilla

Combine the egg whites, Karo, sugar and salt in the top of a double boiler. Place the top over rapidly boiling water and cook, beating constantly with a rotary beater till the frosting stands in peaks. Remove from the heat, add the flavoring and beat well to incorporate it.

This frosting is so old nobody remembers who pioneered the original. My Grandma used to make it in the 1940's.

PEANUT BUTTER FROSTING

Peanut butter frosting
1/3 peanut butter
2/3 cup Karo syrup
Beat together till spreadable. You get about 1 cup frosting with this, so you may want to double or triple the recipe.

VARIATION: add 1 square of semi-sweet baking chocolate that has been melted to make a chocolate peanut butter version.

VARIATION: let a pkg of cream cheese soften to room temperature and beat it into this for a cream cheese peanut butter frosting.

111

OLD TIMEY CORNSTARCH PUDDING

Old timey cornstarch pudding
    3 T cornstarch
    ¼ tsp salt
4 T sugar
3 cups milk
1 tsp vanilla

Sift together the cornstarch, salt and sugar. Add ½ cup milk. Blend until smooth. In a double boiler put the remaining milk and boil till frothy. Gradually pour the milk into the cornstarch mixture, stirring constantly. Return the whole mixture to the heat. Cook stirring constantly till the mixture thickens. Remove the spoon. Cover the double boiler and allow the pudding to cook 25 minutes, stirring often. Remove from the heat. Cool. Add the flavoring, coloring can be added here, if desired. Beat well and pour into individual cups to chill.

Variation: right before removing from the heat toss in some baking chocolate or chocolate chips and stir till the chocolate melts to make chocolate pudding.

MERINGUE

Meringue
3 tsp cold water
1/8 tsp salt
3 egg whites
¼ tsp cream of tartar
6 T sugar
¾ tsp vanilla

Add water and salt to the egg whites. Beat until white and fluffy. Add the cream of tartar. Beat until nearly stiff. Gradually add the sugar, while beating constantly. The vanilla is last to be beaten in. Immediately spread on the pie, or whatever you are using it to top. Be sure to seal around the edges, if you are making pie. If the pie crust was chilled before this step, and if you sealed the edge with meringue it will not pull away from the edges during baking. Bake at 350F 15 minutes, the peaks will be slightly brown.

Variation: you can add a little cocoa to make a chocolate meringue. About ¼ cup should do. Add it after the meringue is stiff.

CHIFFON LAYER CAKE

C hiffon layer cake
2 eggs, separated
1 ½ cups sugar
2 ¼ cups sifted cake flour
½ tsp salt
3 tsp double action baking powder
1/3 cup oil
1 cup milk
1 ½ tsp flavoring, vanilla is the most common

Preheat the oven to 350F. Grease the pans (9-in) generously, and dust with flour. Beat the egg whites till frothy. Gradually beat in ½ cup of the sugar, continue beating till very stiff and glossy. In another bowl, sift the remaining sugar, flour, salt, baking powder. Add oil, ½ the milk, flavoring. Beat 1-minute, medium speed on a mixer. Scrape the sides and bottom of the bowl constantly. Add the remaining milk, egg yolks, beat 1 more minute. Fold in the beaten egg white meringue. Pour into the prepared cake pans. Bake the layers for 25-30 minutes, if doing a sheet cake instead of layers bake it for 35-40 minutes, cupcakes for 18-20 minutes.

Light fluffy frostings do well on these light cakes. The boiled marshmallow frosting is perfect.

CHOCOLATE CHIFFON CAKE

Chocolate chiffon cake
    2 eggs, separated
    1 ½ cups sugar
1 ¾ cups cake flour
¾ tsp baking soda
½ tsp salt
1/3 cup oil
1 cup buttermilk
2 squares semi-sweet baking chocolate, melted
1 tsp rum flavoring
2 tsp instant coffee

Preheat the oven to 350F. Grease and dust with flour the round cake pans for the layers. Beat the egg whites till frothy. Gradually beat in ½ cup of the sugar. Continue beating till stiff and glossy. In another bowl sift together the remaining sugar, flour, baking soda, and salt. Add the oil and ½ of the buttermilk. Beat 1 minute on medium speed. Add the remaining buttermilk, egg yolks, flavoring, chocolate and coffee. Beat 1 more minute. Fold in the egg white mixture and pour it into the cake pans. Bake layers for 30-35 minutes. Bake a sheet cake version for 40-45 minutes. Frost with a light fluffy frosting.

LEMON CRUMBLY CRUNCH

L emon crumbly crunch
½ cup sugar
2 T flour
1/8 tsp salt
1 cup hot water
2 well-beaten eggs
1/3 cup lemon juice
1 ½ tsp lemon peel zest

Combine the sugar, flour and salt. Add the water and mix well. Cook over hot water in a double boiler till it thickens. Stir constantly. Remove from the heat and stir in a small amount of the hot mixture into the eggs. Add the egg mixture back to the hot mixture. Cook over hot water again for 2 minutes, stirring constantly. Add the lemon juice, the zest and continue cooking 1 minute. Remove from the heat. Cool. Make a crumbly mix of: ½ cup softened butter, 1 cup dark brown sugar, add 1 cup flour, ½ tsp salt, 1 cup crunchy cereal, ½ cup shredded coconut. Mix it all till crumbly. Grease a baking pan and put 2/3 of the crumbly mix in the bottom of the pan. Pour the cooked mixture over the crust, and top with the remaining 1/3 of the crumbly mix. Bake at 350F for 40 minutes. Serve with ice cream.

GRANDMA'S APPLE CAKE

Grandma's Apple Cake

1 ¼ cup oil

1 cup molasses

1 ½ cup honey

2 eggs

1 cup whole wheat flour plus 1 ½ cups rolled oats

1 tsp rum flavoring

3 cups thinly sliced apples, granny smith

1 cup black walnuts

1 tsp cinnamon

½ tsp ginger

¼ tsp nutmeg

Blend the oil, honey, molasses, cinnamon, ginger, nutmeg and eggs. Mix in the flour, oats and rum. Fold in the apples, and nuts, the mix will be very stiff. Taste the batter. Molasses and honey will need to be sweeter than you really want the end result, because unlike sugar, the sweetness will partially cook out of the cake. Add more till it's almost too sweet. Bake in a greased 9X13 glass dish for 45 minutes. At 350F

KIMMY'S ORANGE SUGAR COOKIES

K immy's Orange sugar cookies
1 cup butter, soft
2 cups sugar
2 eggs
2 tsp orange flavoring
1 tsp orange zest
3 ½ cups flour
2 ½ tsp baking powder
½ tsp salt

Cream the butter and sugar, add the eggs and the flavoring. Sift together the dry ingredients and add a bit at a time mixing in between. Pinch off small pieces of dough and roll into balls. Place the balls 2 inches apart on the cookie sheet, be sure you grease the cookie sheet first. Dip a small juice glass in granulated sugar and use the bottom to gently mash the cookies to about ¼ inch thick. Bake at 350F for 10-12 minutes till the edges start to brown.

Frosting: small pkg cream cheese, 2 cups powdered sugar, 1 tsp orange flavoring, ½ tsp orange zest, 1/8 cup orange juice. Cream the frosting with all ingredients except the juice. Add the juice a tiny bit at a time just to get a smooth icing. The flavor comes mostly from the flavoring.

PECAN PIE WITH CHOCOLATE

Pecan Pie with chocolate
  1 cup corn syrup
  1 cup dark brown sugar
1/3 tsp salt
1/3 cup melted butter
1 tsp rum flavoring
3 eggs, beaten
1 cup heaping, pecan halves
2 squares semi-sweet baking chocolate, melted

Melt the chocolate in a double boiler and let is stay over warm water. Combine the syrup, sugar, salt, butter, rum and mix. Add the chocolate and mix again. Add the slightly beaten eggs. Pour into a 9-inch pie shell and cover the top with the pecans. Bake at 350F for 45 minutes.

Variation: you can add ½ cup shredded coconut, and chocolate chips as well for a loaded pecan pie.

BROWNIE PIE

B rownie Pie
   1 cup sugar
   2 eggs
1 square unsweetened baking chocolate
1 stick butter
2/3 cup flour, sifted
1 tsp vanilla, or your favorite, rum is nice too
1/3 cup pecans, chopped
Chocolate cookie crumb crust

Beat sugar and butter together, add the eggs. Beat till well blended. Add the flour and blend well, add the melted chocolate, flavoring and nuts. Pour into the crust and bake at 325F for 25 minutes, or until a knife inserted comes out clean. You can bake this in a buttered pan without a crust, but that's up to the cook. Serve warm with ice cream

GRANDMA'S BLACK WALNUT CAKE

Grandma's Black Walnut Cake
1 pkg pecan cake mix
2 cups black walnuts, chopped
1 small box vanilla pudding mix
4 eggs
½ cup melted butter
2 bottles black walnut flavoring
1 cup of water and flavoring mixed
Icing:
1 can sweetened condensed milk
1 ready-made German chocolate frosting
1 cup black walnuts, chopped

Pour 2 bottles of black walnut flavoring and add water to make 1 cup. Pour the flavoring mix and all the other ingredients into the mixer bowl. Beat 2 minutes on medium speed. Bake at 350F in a large buttered and floured baking pan for 50 minutes. As soon as the cake is taken out of the oven pour the sweetened condensed milk onto the hot cake, and poke holes in the cake with a knife. Let the cake cool. Frost it with the German chocolate frosting and top with the remaining black walnuts. Or you can mix the nuts into the frosting before frosting the cake.

ORANGE NUT BREAD

O range Nut Bread
2 T butter, soft
1 cup honey

1 egg

1 T grated orange rind

2 ¾ cups flour

2 ½ tsp baking powder

½ tsp baking soda

½ tsp salt

¾ cup orange juice

½ cup sour cream

1 cup nuts, chopped

1 tsp orange flavoring

Blend the soft butter and honey. Beat the egg, orange rind and sour cream. Add those to the honey mixture. Mix well. Sift the dry ingredients together. Add the orange flavor to the orange juice and stir well. Add the dry ingredients alternating with the orange juice. Add the nuts and blend well. Bake in a greased loaf pan at 325F one hour and 10 minutes.

Cream cheese spread to use on the orange loaf:

2 pkg cream cheese, softened

½ tsp orange flavor

½ cup honey

Blend well and taste for sweetness. Add honey if it needs it. And blend well.

ORANGE CREAM CHEESE FROSTING

Orange Cream Cheese Frosting
 1 pkg. cream cheese, softened
 2 cups powdered sugar
1 tsp orange juice
½ tsp orange flavoring
½ tsp grated orange peel
Blend the soft cream cheese and the sifted sugar. Add the orange juice, flavoring and peel. Blend well, and taste it. Use on cooled cakes, or on orange loaf bread, recipe in this book

LEMONADE PIE

L emonade Pie
1 can frozen lemonade, thawed out
1 can sweetened condensed milk
1 9-oz frozen whipped topping, thawed out

Stir in the sweetened condensed milk, and the lemonade. Fold in the whipped topping and pour into 2 graham cracker crusts. Refrigerate to chill. You can do this with any frozen juice concentrate. Orange juice is popular the raspberry lime is great.

OLD TIMEY APPLE PIE

Old timey Apple Pie
1 egg, large, beaten
1 ¼ cups sugar
1 stick melted butter
1 tsp cinnamon
¼ tsp salt
1 ½ cups grated coarsely tart apple
1 unbaked pie shell, deep dish

Lay the grated apple in the crust. Top the apples with pats of butter, and sprinkle cinnamon over them. Mix all the other ingredients together and pour over the apples. Bake at 350F for 35 minutes.

CREME DE MENTHE MARSHMALLOW PIE

Crème de Menthe Marshmallow Pie
Chocolate crust, freeze it
1 bag marshmallows
½ cup crème de menthe
½ pint heavy cream
Chocolate chips

Beat the heavy cream into stiff whipped cream. Melt 24 of the marshmallows and mix the crème de menthe into the melted marshmallows. Fold in the whipped cream, pour it or spoon it into the frozen pie crust. Garnish with the chocolate chips. You could use Andes mints broken into pieces instead. Chill the pie for a few hours before serving.

KEY LIME PIE

Key Lime Pie
    4 large limes, juiced
    1 can sweetened condensed milk
1 cup Heavy cream
¼ cup sugar
1 cup chocolate shavings, you can grate 1 bar baking chocolate to get this
1 graham cracker crust
2 T grated lime zest
Combine the zest, the lime juice and the condensed milk. Mix well and set aside. Beat the heavy cream till peaks form, add the sugar in while beating, till stiff peaks form. Fold the lime juice mixture with the whipped cream. Spoon it into the pie crust, and top with chocolate shavings. Chill several hours.

PECAN CRUST SWEET POTATO PIE

Pecan crust sweet potato pie
For the crust:
¾ cups pecans, chopped fine
1/3 cup dark brown sugar, packed
2-3 T soft butter
Blend together to form a crumbly dough, press into a greased pie pan to form a crust on the bottom and sides.
2/3 cup dark brown sugar, packed
2 eggs, beaten frothy
1 cup cooked sweet potatoes, mashed
1 T flour
½ tsp cinnamon
½ tsp ginger
¼ tsp nutmeg
1 cup light cream
Marshmallows to top at the end of the baking time
Mix the ingredients gently with a blender on low speed. Pour into the pecan crust and bake at 350F 50 minutes or until a knife inserted comes out clean. Top with marshmallows and pop into the oven till the marshmallows melt and start to toast. Remove from the oven and chill.

ORANGE SLICE CAKE

Orange Slice Cake (this is an old classic; we've all forgotten who invented it)

    Cream until light:

1 cup butter

2 cups sugar

Beat in 4 eggs, one at a time

Add ½ pkg coconut

Add:

½ cup buttermilk

1 tsp baking soda

In a large mixing bowl, stir to well coat each piece:

3 ½ cups flour

1 lb. dates, chopped

1 lb. candy orange slices, chopped

2 cups pecans, chopped

The reason you coat the stuff with flour is so it stays suspended in the cake and doesn't all fall to the bottom of the cake during baking. The mixture will be stiff, so you will mix it with your hands. Mix everything together at this point. Pour it all into a well-greased and floured 9X13 baking pan. Bake at 250F for 2 ½-3 hours.

    Combine

1 cup orange juice and 2 cups powdered sugar, pour over the hot cake. Chill overnight in the pan it baked in.

NO BAKE CHERRY CHEESE PIE

No Bake Cherry Cheese pie
  1 graham cracker crust
  1 8-oz pkg. cream cheese, softened
1 can sweetened condensed milk
1/3 cup lemon juice
1 tsp vanilla
1 can cherry pie filling

In a bowl, beat the cream cheese to fluffy. Add the sweetened condensed milk and blend well. Stir in the lemon juice, and vanilla. Mix well. Pour into the crust, chill 3 hours. Top with the cherries before serving.

KIMMY'S ALMOND COOKIES

Kimmy's Almond cookies
    1 small pkg. cream cheese
    ½ cup butter, soft

2 cup sugar

1 cup brown sugar

1 can almond paste

2 eggs

3 tsp almond flavoring

3 ½ cups flour

2 tsp baking powder

½ tsp salt

1 large bag sliced almonds

Cream the butter, cream cheese, sugars, and almond paste together. Add the eggs and flavoring. Sift the dry ingredients together and add gradually. Blend smooth. The almonds are not part of the dry ingredients. Make balls from the dough, mash them with a small juice glass dipped in sugar to about ¼ inch thick. Bake at 350F for 10-12 minutes. The edges will start to brown when done. Remove from the cookie sheet. Make the frosting and add an almond or two on top of the frosting.

Frosting: 1 small pkg cream cheese, 1 cup powdered sugar, 2 tsp almond flavoring Blend well to smooth consistency. Add a bit of milk if needed to make it smooth.

KIMMY'S CHRISTMAS BROWNIES

K immy's Christmas Brownies
2 cups sugar
2 eggs, slightly beaten
¼ tsp salt
½ cup flour
½ cup pecans, chopped
½ tsp peppermint flavoring
4 squares semi-sweet chocolate, or 1 pkg choc chips
¼ cup butter

Melt the chocolate with the butter, add in the other ingredients and blend well. Pour the batter into a 9X13 baking pan and bake at 350F for 35-40 minutes or until a knife inserted comes out clean.

Frosting: 1 small pkg cream cheese, 2 squares semi-sweet baking chocolate, melted, ½ cup powdered sugar, ½ tsp peppermint flavoring. Blend all together till smooth and spreading consistency. If its too stiff add some milk 1 T at a time to loosen it up.

You can add crushed peppermint candy to the frosting too or use it as a garnish.

KIMMY'S CHOCOLATE AND LACE COOKIES

K immy's chocolate and lace cookies
½ cup butter, melted in a saucepan
Stir in:

½ cup sugar

1/3 cup flour

¼ tsp salt

1 cup quick oats

2 T milk

Mix well. Drop by spoonfuls onto a greased and floured cookie sheet. These spread, so keep 3 inches between them. Bake at 350F for 7 minutes, or till edges brown. Remove after 1 minute from the cookie sheet. They should be very flexible. If they are too stiff reheat to soften them. Let them cool.

Melt 1 pkg. chocolate chips and 2 T butter in a double boiler. Turn the heat to low. Paint the chocolate on the top of a lace cookie and top it with another cookie making a sandwich of chocolate and lace. If you have a large family, you will want to double or triple the recipe and get the kiddos involved.

For a Christmas version add 1/8 tsp peppermint to the chocolate

KARO PECAN PIE

Karo pecan pie
   3 eggs, beaten
   1 cup Karo
1 cup sugar
2 T butter, melted
1 tsp vanilla or rum
2 cups pecans
1–9-inch pie shell

In a large bowl, stir eggs, Karo, sugar, butter and flavoring till well blended. Stir in the pecans. Pour into the pie shell and bake at 350F for 50-55 minutes. A knife inserted will come out clean.

134

SUPER EASY FROZEN MINT PIE

Super easy frozen mint pie
    1 Oreo crust
    1 can sweetened condensed milk

1. ½ tsp peppermint extract

A few drops of green food coloring
1-pint heavy whipping cream
1 box Andes mints, chopped
In a large mixer combine whipping cream, beat till peaks form, add the sweetened condensed milk, peppermint and food coloring, beat till well combined. Fold in ½ the Andes mints. Pour into the pie crust. Sprinkle with the remaining Andes mints to garnish. Chill for 6 hours.

KIMMY'S CHOCOLATE MINT CHEESECAKE (FOR DIABETICS)

K immy's chocolate mint cheesecake (for diabetics)
1-chocolate crusts
3-8oz. pkg. cream cheese
2 cups stevia, for baking type
2-eggs
¼ tsp peppermint extract, you can use up to ½ tsp
2 bars semi-sweet baking chocolate

Cream together all the above except the chocolate. Melt 1 of the whole bars of baking chocolate in a double boiler or microwave, mix it into the cheesecake mixture. You will use 4 pieces of the other chocolate bar to melt and drizzle over the cheesecake after it comes out of the oven. Pour the cheesecake mixture into the 2 crusts. Bake at 325F for 35-40 minutes or until a toothpick inserted comes out clean. Drizzle the melted 4 pieces of chocolate over the cheesecake and chill for 4 hours.

KIMMY'S EASY CHOCOLATE CHIP CHEESECAKE

K immy's easy chocolate chip cheesecake
2 8-oz. pkg. cream cheese
½ cup sugar
2 eggs
½ tsp rum
½ cup chocolate chips

Mix all the ingredients together well. Pour the batter into the crust and bake at 350F for 40 minutes. A toothpick inserted should come out clean. Chill for 4 hours.

KIMMY'S PUMPKIN PIE

Kimmy's pumpkin pie
1 large can of pumpkin puree
1 can sweetened condensed milk
2 eggs
1 tsp cinnamon
½ tsp ginger
½ tsp nutmeg
2 deep dish crusts

Combine all the ingredients and pour into the 2 pie crusts. Bake at 425F for 15 minutes, then reduce the heat to 350F for 35-40 minutes or till a knife inserted comes out clean. You should cover the edges of the crust to keep them from browning too much.

HOPE'S PUMPKIN PIE VARIATION FOR DIABETICS

Hope's pumpkin pie variation for diabetics
1large can of pumpkin puree
1 can evaporated milk
1/3 cup honey
4T unsweetened applesauce
1 tsp cinnamon
½ tsp ginger
½ tsp nutmeg
2 deep dish pie crusts

Mix all the ingredients above and pour into 2 deep dish pie crusts. Bake at 425F for 15 minutes then reduce the oven temperature to 350F for 35-40 minutes or until a knife inserted comes out clean.

HONEY IS LOW GLYCEMIC INDEX. We leave out the eggs in this one in favor of unsweetened applesauce because Hope has egg allergies. You can do this too for vegans.

APPLE PIE

Apple Pie
    2cups thinly sliced tart apples
    1 cup dark brown sugar, packed

¼ cup water

1T lemon juice

¼ cup flour

2T sugar

1 tsp vanilla

3 T butter

Pastry for crust

Mix the apples, brown sugar, water and lemon juice in a saucepan. Cover and cook till the apples are just starting to be tender. Mix the flour sugar and a pinch of salt. Stir it into the apple mixture in the saucepan. Cook, stirring constantly, until the mixture thickens and boils, continue cooking for 2 minutes. Remove from the heat. Stir in the vanilla and butter. Cool to room temperature. Preheat the oven to 425F. prepare the pastry. Turn the apple mixture into the pastry lined pan and cover with the remaining pastry. Cut slits in the top pastry to vent, seal the edges of the upper and lower pastry. You will cover the edges of the pie with foil to keep them from going too dark in the baking process. Bake 40-45 minutes.

Pastry:

2/3 cup plus 2T butter

2 cups flour

½ tsp salt

4-5 T freezing cold water

Cut the butter into the flour with a pastry blender or 2 knives till it resembles crumbles. Should look like peas. Sprinkle in the water and mash with a fork till all the flour is moistened and dough is cleaning sides of the bowl. Gather the pastry into a ball, divide the ball in ½. Shape each ½ into a flat round shape and roll in flour till the circle is 2 inches larger than the inverted pie pan. Fold the one circle into 4ths. And unfold it inside the pie pan, easing it into the corners of the bottom of the pie pan. The top circle of pastry goes over the filling after you put it in the bottom pastry.

KIMMY'S CHOCOLATE COCONUT ALMOND CHEESECAKE

Kimmy's chocolate coconut almond cheesecake
1 chocolate cookie crust
4 8-oz. pkg. cream cheese
3 eggs
1 cup sugar
1 pkg. shredded coconut
1 12-oz. pkg. chocolate chips, melted
½ cup slivered almonds
1 tsp vanilla
½ cup semi-sweet chocolate chips plus ½ cup toasted coconut

Beat the cream cheese, eggs and sugar at medium speed till fluffy. Stir in the melted chocolate chips and beat to blend. Fold in the almonds, coconut and flavoring. Pour the cheesecake mixture into the pie crust. Bake at 350F for 50 minutes, or until a knife inserted comes out clean. Melt the remaining semi-sweet chocolate chips and drizzle over the cheesecake and sprinkle the toasted coconut on top before chilling. Chill 8 hours.

FUDGE FILLED CHEESECAKE

F udge filled cheesecake
½ cup butter, softened
1/3 cup sugar
1 tsp vanilla
1 cup flour
2/3 cup pistachios, chopped fine

Beat the butter at medium speed till creamy. Add the sugar and beat well. Gradually add the flour on low speed till blended. Stir in 1 tsp vanilla and the chopped pistachios. Press the dough into a pie pan to form a crust. Bake at 350F 12-15 minutes till golden. Let cool.

4 8oz. pkgs. of cream cheese
1 ½ cups sugar
1 tsp vanilla
4 large eggs
1 12oz. chocolate chips

Beat the cream cheese till light and fluffy. Gradually add the sugar, beating well. Add the eggs one at a time, beating between them, just until the yellow disappears. Stir in the remaining vanilla and pour ½ the batter into the pie crust. Cover the batter completely with the chocolate chips. Add the remaining batter over the chocolate chips. Bake at 350F for 50 minutes till set. Cool for an hour before serving.

EASY FUDGE

E asy fudge
   3 cups semi-sweet chocolate chips
   1 can sweetened condensed milk
Dash of salt

1 cup pecans, chopped small

2 T rum

In a heavy saucepan melt the chocolate chips with the sweetened condensed milk and the salt over low heat. Remove from the heat and stir in the nuts and rum. Grease an 8-inch baking pan and put wax paper in the bottom. Butter the paper top. Pour the fudge in the pan and chill till it sets up. Cut into squares and turn the pan out onto a tray, peel the wax paper off the fudge.

DOUBLE CHOCOLATE AND
BUTTERSCOTCH CHIP COOKIES

Double chocolate and butterscotch chip cookies
  1 box chocolate cake mix
  ½ cup oil or melted butter
2 eggs
2 cups butterscotch chips
2 cups chocolate chips
1 cup pecans chopped small
Combine the cake mix and butter and eggs in a bowl, mix well. Stir in the butterscotch and chocolate chips and nuts. Drop by spoonfuls onto a cookie sheet and bake at 350F for 8-10 minutes.

PECAN DATE CAKE

Pecan date cake
    2 tsp baking soda
    1 ½ cup boiling water
4 cups chopped dates
1 ½ cup butter, soft
2 cups sugar
8 eggs
4 cups flour
2 tsp baking powder
1 cup pecans, chopped

Put the baking soda in the boiling water. Add the chopped dates and let soak for 20 minutes. Cream the butter with the sugar. Add the eggs one at a time beating well. Sift the flour and baking powder together and blend into the beaten mixture. Add the date mixture, then the flour mixture. Add the nuts and stir well. Pour into a greased and floured tube pan bake at 350F for 1 hour and 15 minutes.

CHOCOLATE ORANGE GANACHE FROSTING

Chocolate orange ganache frosting
1 cup heavy cream
1 ½ cups semi-sweet chocolate chips
1 T butter
2 tsp orange extract

Heat the cream to boiling in a heavy saucepan. Add the chocolate chips, let it sit 4 minutes. Whisk until the chips are melted. Whisk again and pour onto the cake or whatever you are frosting. If you want to use this inside candy refrigerate it first.

CHOCOLATE TRUFFLE CAKE
(FLOURLESS)

C hocolate truffle cake (flourless chocolate cake)
      1 ½ cups butter, soft (2 ½ sticks)
      ¾ cup cocoa

1 cup sugar

1T flour

2 tsp rum

4 eggs, separated

1 cup cold heavy whipping cream (1/2 pint)

1 square semi-sweet baking chocolate grated into chocolate curls

Preheat the oven to 400F. Grease the bottom of a springform pan. Melt the butter over low heat in a heavy saucepan. Add the cocoa and the sugar and stir well. Remove from the heat and allow to cool slightly. Stir in the flour and the rum and add the egg yolks one at a time beating in between. Beat the egg whites in a bowl with a T of sugar and keep beating till peaks start to hold shape. Gradually fold in the chocolate mixture. Spoon the mixture into the pan. Bake it at 400F for 16-18 minutes, the edge will firm up, but the center will be soft. Cool completely the cake will sink in the middle as it cools. Remove the sidewalls of the spring form pan. Chill for 6 hours. Let the cake warm up to room temperature before serving. You can garnish with whipped cream and chocolate curls.

. . .

NOTE: this is often called "flourless chocolate cake" in restaurants. It is a famous dessert in Italy, by another name, but I can't spell it in Italian.

TRIPLE LAYER CHEESECAKE

Triple layer cheesecake
    3 8-oz. pkgs. cream cheese
    ¾ cup sugar
3 eggs
1/3 cup sour cream
3 T flour
1 tsp vanilla
1 tsp rum
1 tsp butter flavoring
¼ tsp salt
1 cup semi-sweet chocolate chips, melted
1 cup butterscotch chips melted

Preheat the oven to 350F. Prepare a chocolate cookie crumb crust by using cookie crumbs and melted butter to make the crust. Beat the softened cream cheese and sugar in a bowl till smooth. Add the eggs, sour cream, flour and salt. Beat until blended. Separate the cheesecake mixture into thirds. Mix 1/3 into the melted chocolate, add the vanilla and beat till smooth. Add 1/3 to the butterscotch and beat till smooth. Add the rum and butter flavoring to the last 1/3 and beat to incorporate it. Pour the butterscotch layer into the chocolate crust. Pour the butter rum layer over the butterscotch layer and pour the chocolate layer over the butter rum layer. Bake in the oven at 350F for 55-60 minutes or until a toothpick inserted comes out clean. You can melt the same type of chocolate and butterscotch chips in a double boiler to detail the top of the cheesecake if you want to make it pretty. Or you could just add some whipped cream and chocolate shavings.

VARIATION: if you can't find chocolate cookie crumbs you can use any flavor mixed with cocoa. Graham crackers will work. 1 ½ cups cookie crumbs, ¼ cup cocoa, and butter, melted and mixed into the mixture. Taste it and add sugar if needed.

MOCHA FUDGE CAKE

Mocha fudge cake
1 ¼ cup butter (2 ½ sticks)
¾ cup special dark cocoa
4 eggs
¼ tsp salt
1 tsp rum
¼ cup instant coffee
2 cups sugar
1 cup flour
1 cup pecans, chopped small

Preheat the oven to 350F. Butter two 9-inch round cake pans. Line the bottoms of the pans with parchment paper, butter the top of the paper. Melt the butter sticks in a saucepan, remove from the heat and add the cocoa and instant coffee. Stir well to blend. Cool slightly. Beat the eggs in a large mixing bowl till frothy. Add the salt and rum. Gradually add the sugar, beating well. Add the cooled chocolate mixture. Fold in the flour and nuts. Pour the cake batter into the two pans. Bake 20-25 minutes till a toothpick inserted into the middle comes out clean. Cool 5 minutes. Gently flip the cake onto wire racks to cool. Place the rack over the cake pan and gently roll it over. The parchment paper should make this easy. After the cake cools gently remove the parchment paper. Frost with the creamy mocha frosting.

Creamy mocha frosting:

1 ½ cups heavy whipping cream, 1/3 cup dark brown sugar, packed, ¼ cup instant coffee, ¼ cup cocoa. In a saucepan melt the brown sugar, coffee, cocoa and 3T butter set aside. In a bowl beat the whipping cream till peaks form. Gently pour in the coffee mixture beating the whole time till its well blended. Use for frosting the mocha cake.

Chocolate raspberry cheesecake

3 8-oz. pkgs. Cream cheese

¾ cup sugar

3 eggs

1/3 cup sour cream

3 T flour

1 tsp vanilla

¼ tsp salt

2 cups semi-sweet chocolate chips, melted

1 ½ cups frozen raspberries, cover with 1/8 cup sugar and refrigerate overnight

1 chocolate cookie crumb crust

Preheat the oven to 350F. Beat the cream cheese and sugar in a bowl on medium speed till smooth. Add the eggs, flour, sour cream, vanilla and salt. Split the cheesecake batter into 2 equal parts. In one half of the mixture fold in and mix the chocolate till well blended. In the other ½ beat in the raspberries you chilled overnight, saving a small amount of it to top the cheesecake later. Blend well. The berries will mash and color the cheesecake. Pour the berry flavor cheesecake batter into the crust, top the berry layer with the chocolate layer. Bake at 350F for 55-60 minutes or until a toothpick inserted in the middle comes out clean. Allow the cheesecake to cool. Top with the remaining raspberries. Chill for 6 hours.

ESPRESSO CHOCOLATE CHEESECAKE

Espresso chocolate cheesecake
1 chocolate cookie crust
4 8-oz. pkgs. cream cheese
2/3 cup sugar
1 1/3 cups semi-sweet chocolate chips
3 eggs
1/3 cup heavy cream
1 T instant espresso powder (used in baking not drinking)
¼ tsp cinnamon
¼ cup cocoa

Preheat the oven to 350F. Melt 1 cup of the chocolate chips in a small saucepan over low heat, stir constantly. Combine cream cheese, and sugar in a large bowl beat on medium speed till smooth. Add the eggs, cream, espresso powder, cocoa and cinnamon, beat at low speed till well blended. Add the melted chocolate, mix to blend. Beat for 2 minutes on medium speed. Spoon the cheesecake batter into the crust. Bake at 350F for 55 minutes or until a toothpick inserted in the center comes out clean. Cool completely before garnishing with espresso cream.

Espresso cream: ½ cup cold heavy whipping cream, 2 T powdered sugar, 1 T espresso powder, 2 tsp cocoa. Beat the whipping cream till peaks form, add the sugar, espresso and cocoa and beat again till all is blended well.

HERSHEY'S KISSES COOKIES

Hershey's kisses cookies
1 cup butter, soft
2/3 cup sugar
1 tsp rum
1 2/3 cups flour
¼ cup cocoa
1 cup pecans, chopped small
Hershey's kisses, unwrap them
1 cup powdered sugar sifted with ¼ cup cocoa to roll the cookies in after baking

Beat the butter, sugar and rum together in a bowl till creamy. Stir together the flour and cocoa, gradually add the flour mixture to the creamy mixture, beat well to blend it. Add the pecans and blend well. Refrigerate the dough to firm it up. Preheat the oven to 350F. When the dough is chilled take it out of the fridge and mash it around the Hershey kisses, completely covering the kiss and forming a ball shaped cookie. Place on an ungreased cookie sheet. Bake 10-12 minutes to set the cookie dough. Cool for 1 minute before trying to remove from the cookie sheet. Roll the warm cookies in the powdered cocoa mix and set on a plate to cool completely.

HOT WATER PIE CRUST

Hot water pie crust
1/2 cup butter flavored Crisco
¼ cup boiling water
2 cups flour
¼ tsp baking powder
½ tsp salt

Place the Crisco in a bowl and pour in the boiling water and salt. Beat till smooth and creamy. Sift the flour and baking powder into the Crisco mixture and stir with a fork till it leaves the sides of the bowl. Chill till it becomes firm. Roll out the chilled dough as normal for pie.

Variation: add 2 T lemon juice to the boiling water for a lemon flavored crust.

GREEN TOMATO PIE

Green tomato pie
2 cups green (unripe) tomatoes, chopped
½ cup chopped dates
¼ tsp ground cloves
½ cup dark brown sugar, packed
1 tsp salt
1 tsp cinnamon
1T vinegar
1 T lemon zest
1/8 tsp nutmeg

Mix all the ingredients together. Line a pie tin with pie crust. Pour the mixture into the crust. And top the pie with a top crust, seal the edges. Dot the top with lots of butter pats and sprinkle on brown sugar. Bake at 350F for 20-30 minutes.

CANDIED APPLE PIE

C andied apple pie
    ½ cup butter
    1cup dark brown sugar
1cup sifted flour

7-tart apples

Slice the apples and lay them in a pie pan. Cream the butter, sugar and flour together and pour it over the apples. Bake at 300F for 50 minutes.

STRAWBERRY RHUBARB PIE

S trawberry rhubarb pie
  I cup sugar
  ¼ tsp salt
1/8 tsp nutmeg
2 T quick tapioca
¼ cup orange juice
3 cups sliced rhubarb
I cup sliced strawberries
I T butter

Combine the sugar, salt, nutmeg, tapioca, orange juice and rhubarb. Place in a 9-inch pie pan lined with the orange crust. The orange crust is in this book. Top the mixture with the strawberries. Dot the whole top with butter pieces. Roll out another orange crust and slice it into strips to lattice over the pie top. Seal and flute the edges. Bake at 450F for 10 minutes, then reduce the oven temperature to 350F for 30 minutes.

FRIED APPLE PIES

Fried apple pies
    1cup flour
    6T baked apples, chopped
¼ cup butter, slices
½ tsp salt
Cold water

Sift the flour and salt together in a bowl. Work in the butter, using a pastry blender. Add the water a bit at a time to form a dough. Roll out circles of dough about 5 inches across. Spoon the baked apples into the center of the dough. Fold over the dough and seal the edges. Fry in oil. Lay on a paper towel lined tray and sprinkle with cinnamon sugar.

156

CINNAMON BAKED APPLES

Cinnamon baked apples

1. large apples cored and sliced

1T lemon juice
¼ cup dark brown sugar
1T sugar
2 tsp cinnamon
2 tsp cornstarch
2T butter

Preheat the oven to 350F. Lay the sliced apples into a baking pan. Mix together the lemon juice, brown sugar, sugar, cinnamon and cornstarch. Spread evenly onto the apples. Top with the butter, cut into small pieces. Cover with aluminum foil and bake at 350F for 30-40 minutes. You will stir these often while they bake. Remove from the oven. Chill or serve hot with ice cream.

COCONUT PIE SHELL

Coconut pie shell
  1 12-oz. pkg shredded coconut
  1/4lb. butter

Preheat oven to 350F. Place the coconut in a bowl. Add the butter. Knead the two together. You want it mixed well. Gently work the mixture into a pie pan to form a crust. Bake for 10-15 minutes to set. If you want more of a toasted coconut flavor bake a bit longer smelling till it seems right. Remove from heat and allow to cool.

TOASTED COCONUT PIE

Toasted coconut pie
    1 ½ cups toasted coconut
    1 coconut crust (in this book)
3 eggs, beaten
1 ½ cups sugar
½ cup butter, melted
1T lemon juice
1T almond extract
½ cup almond paste

Preheat the oven to 350F. In a large bowl combine the coconut, eggs, sugar, butter, lemon juice, almond paste and almond extract. Mix well. Pour into the coconut crust. Bake in the oven at 350F 45-50 minutes. It will be golden. You can protect the edges of the pie with aluminum foil to keep it from being burnt. You can serve it warm or chilled.

COCONUT PIE OLD FASHIONED STYLE

Coconut pie old fashioned style
    1 coconut crust (recipe in this section)
    1 ½ cups sugar
½ cup butter, soft
2 eggs
½ tsp salt
¼ cup flour
½ cup heavy cream
1 ½ cups toasted coconut flakes

Preheat oven to 350F. Beat the butter, sugar, eggs, and salt to a nice lemon color. Add in the flour, blend well. Beat in the cream. Fold in the toasted coconut. Pour into the coconut crust. Bake for 1 hour. Cover the crust edges with foil during the baking. Let cool.

CHOCOLATE COCONUT PIE

Chocolate coconut pie
    1 cup flour
    ¼ cup cocoa
1 cup powdered sugar
½ tsp salt
¾ cup butter, softened

Sift together the flour, cocoa, sugar and salt. Work the butter into the mixture to form a dough. Roll out the dough and line a pie pan with it. This will be the crust for the pie.

Filling:
½ cup heavy whipping cream
8-oz. mascarpone cheese
¼ cup powdered sugar
1 tsp coconut extract
1 tsp almond flavoring
1 ¼ toasted coconut flakes
¼ cup sliced almonds

Topping:
¼ cup heavy whipping cream
4-oz. semi-sweet baking chocolate, chopped

Bake the pie crust we made at 350F for 10 minutes to set it. Whip the whipping cream till peaks form. About 2-3 minutes. Set aside. Whip the mascarpone cheese, powdered sugar, flavorings, on medium till combined well. Fold in the coconut and blend. Spread the filling into the pie crust. Top with the sliced almonds and chill for the topping bring the heavy cream to a boil on the stove. Boil for around 2 minutes, stirring constantly. Remove from heat and add the chocolate pieces. Stir till the chocolate is melted and the topping is smooth and well mixed. Let the topping sit to thicken. When it's an icing consistency top the chilled pie with the topping, smoothing it out as evenly as possible. Return to the fridge to chill.

GINGER SNAPS

Ginger snaps
    ¾ cup Crisco or butter
    1 cup sugar
¼ cup molasses
1 egg
2 cups flour
¼ tsp salt
2 tsp baking soda
1 tsp ginger
1 tsp cinnamon
½ tsp cloves

Cream shortening and sugar together. Add the molasses and egg and beat well. Sift the flour with the other dry ingredients. Add the dry blend to the sugar mixture. Mix well. Roll the batter into ball cookies and dip in sugar. Place the balls 2 inches apart on a greased cookie sheet. Bake at 350F for 12-14 minutes. Makes 5-6 dozen.

COFFEE FUDGE

Coffee fudge
1 cup strong coffee
3 cups sugar
½ cup heavy cream
1/8 tsp salt
2 T butter
½ tsp rum
1 cup pecans, chopped

Put coffee, sugar, salt and cream in a heavy saucepan stir to blend well. Cover and cook to a boil. Remove the lid, add the butter. Cook on medium heat to the soft ball stage. Remove from the heat, add the rum. Allow the mixture to cool. Beat until light in color, smooth and creamy. Add the nuts, beat until it loses its shine. Pour into a buttered baking pan and chill.

PEPPERMINT DIVINITY

Peppermint divinity
    3 cups sugar
    1 cup boiling water
1 cup corn syrup
3 egg whites beaten till stiff peaks form
½ tsp peppermint
Pinch of salt

In a heavy saucepan combine the sugar, water and corn syrup. Cook on the stove on low heat till the soft ball stage (34F). Pour the hot syrup over the egg whites, beating the whole time to blend them. Continue to beat to thicken the mixture. Add the peppermint. Pour into a buttered baking dish and chill till firm. Cut into squares to serve.

Variation you can add nuts with the peppermint. Or you could add candy that has been crushed or chopped.

PECAN PRALINE CHEESECAKE

Pecan praline cheesecake
Praline part:
1 ½ cups sugar
1 ½ cups brown sugar
¼ tsp salt
1cup half and half
6T salted butter
1 tsp vanilla
2 cups pecan pieces

In a heavy saucepan combine the sugars, salt, half and half and butter. Cook over medium heat, till the sugars dissolve and it comes to a boil. Continue cooking till your candy thermometer is at 235F, the soft ball stage. Stir in the vanilla and pecans and beat with a wood spoon till it isn't glossy. Set this aside by putting it in the top of a double boiler and hot water in the bottom, so it doesn't set up, and make the cheesecake part.

Cheesecake part:
4 8-oz. pkgs cream cheese, softened to room temperature
¾ cup sugar
3 eggs
1/3 cup heavy cream
3 T flour
1 tsp butter flavoring

¼ tsp salt

1 graham cracker crust

Beat the softened cream cheese and sugar together till smooth. Add the eggs, cream, flour and salt. Beat until blended. Mix in the butter flavoring. Blend well. Pour ½ the praline mixture into the crust. Pour the cheesecake batter into the crust and pour the remaining praline mixture on top of the cheesecake. Use a butter knife to swirl the topping into the cheesecake. Bake at 350F for 45-50 minutes or until a toothpick inserted into the center comes out clean. Chill a few hours before serving.

SOUR CREAM FUDGE

Sour cream fudge
    3 cups brown sugar
    1 cup sour cream
Pinch of salt
¼ cup butter
1 tsp rum
1 cup pecan pieces

Combine the sugar and sour cream in a heavy saucepan and cook to 240F. basically the soft ball stage. Remove from the heat and add the salt and butter, beat until the mixture begins to get grainy. Stir in the rum and nuts. Pour into a buttered pan and chill.

EASY ALMOND COOKIES

E asy almond cookies
1 lb. butter
2 cups powdered sugar
2 cups finely ground almonds
3 cups flour
3 tsp almond flavoring

Cream the butter and sugar together. Work in the other ingredients. Drop by spoonfuls onto a cookie sheet and bake at 350F for 12-14 minutes. Dip the cookies in powdered sugar while warm. Set onto a tray to cool. You can also put the warm cookies on wax paper and sift the sugar onto them.

NUT CRISPS

Nut crisps
>   1 cup brown sugar
>   1 egg

1 T butter

2 heaping T flour

Pinch of salt

1 cup chopped nuts

Mix the sugar, butter and flour. Add the egg and nuts. Drop spoonfuls onto a cookie sheet and bake at 350F 15-18 minutes. These will stick to the pan, so remove them from the cookie sheet quickly after baking.

OLD SOUTHERN GINGERBREAD

Old southern gingerbread
  1/2 cup butter
  ½ cup sugar

1 cup molasses

2 eggs

2 cups flour

1 tsp baking soda

1 tsp ginger

1 tsp cinnamon

½ cup buttermilk

Add the baking soda to the buttermilk and set aside. Cream the butter and sugar. Add the molasses and eggs to the sugar, beating well after each egg. Sift the dry ingredients that are left together and add them alternating with the milk, back and forth while beating. Bake at 350F for about 20 minutes and test with a toothpick for doneness.

SOUR CREAM LEMON CAKE

Sour cream lemon cake
>   2 eggs
>   1 cup sugar

1 cup sour cream

¼ tsp salt

1T lemon juice

2T grated lemon zest

2 cups flour

1 tsp baking powder

2/3 tsp baking soda

Beat the eggs. Add the sugar beat well. Add all the other ingredients. Blend well. Pour into a greased and floured baking pan and bake at 350F for 30 minutes, then check with a toothpick for doneness.

Lemon frosting: 1 pkg. cream cheese, softened to room temperature. 2 tsp lemon juice. ½ cup sugar. Beat the sugar and the cream cheese till smooth. Add the lemon juice. Mix well and taste it. If it needs more lemon juice add it and beat again till you are happy with the taste. Garnish with grated lemon peel.

CANDIED ORANGE PEEL

C andied orange peel
2 cups sugar
1 cup water
¼ cup corn syrup
Salt
Orange peels

Remove all orange and white inner layer of peels. Cut the peel in quarters. Place the peels in a saucepan and cover with cold water. Add 1 tsp salt for each 2 whole oranges. Bring to a boil and cook for 30 minutes. Drain and cover with fresh hot water, no salt this time. Let boil another 30 minutes. If its not tender, repeat the process till it is tender. When the peel can be pierced with a toothpick, drain and cut into the desired sizes. Make a syrup of the sugar, water and corn syrup. If the peel is cold use the syrup cold. If the peel is hot, use the syrup hot. Bring back to a boil and boil till nearly all the syrup is absorbed by the peels. The peel will become clear. Drain and roll in sugar, place on wax paper to cool and dry. Seal into glass jars for storage.

MINTED CHRISTMAS NUTS

Minted Christmas nuts
1 cup sugar
½ cup water
1 T light corn syrup
1/8 tsp salt
6 marshmallows
½ tsp peppermint extract
3 drops oil of peppermint
3 cups pecans, broken into pieces

Cook together slowly sugar, water, corn syrup and salt. Remove from heat just before the 235F stage. Add marshmallows and stir until they are melted. Add the flavoring and nuts, stirring in circles till every nut is coated and the mixture hardens. Cool the nuts on waxed paper. Store in a glass jar.

CANDIED NUTS

C andied nuts
1 cup sugar
1/3 cup water
1 T butter
1 tsp maple flavoring
2 cups pecans, halved
Pinch of salt

Boil the water and sugar, stir occasionally. When it forms a thread, turn off the heat and add the butter, nuts, maple and salt. Don't overcook we want this creamy like pralines.

AUTHOR BIO

Author Bio:

Kimberley, Hope and Faith are all cooks from a long line of cooks. They live on the southwestern edge of the area of the southern US commonly called Appalachia. The Smokey Mountain range is practically in their back yard. The culture of Appalachia is based around independence in all things including learning to cook. Crafting and making things from the plants and animals is a part of the lifestyle as well. We hope you enjoy the rather southern personality of the dishes shared in this book, and we hope you also check out the other books in the series.

LIVING IN PEACE

Living in the Bible Belt comes with a responsibility to share the wonderful gift of faith that we have been blessed with. If you find your life difficult as you struggle alone against the tide of adversity, you may want to consider asking the God of the universe to be your companion along the way. We have had Him heal our family members when they were injured or sick. We have had Him open doors to opportunities we normally wouldn't have had. We have seen Him protect us in situations that were normally so dangerous the people in those situations would die without His constant care and protection. God sent His son Jesus into the world so that we could have life. And that that life could be abundant. With Jesus we no longer struggle alone, we have ever present help in a friend who sticks closer than a brother. We have a savior and a deliverer. You can have Him too by praying for Him to be in your life. The Bible says:

"That if thou shalt confess with thy mouth the Lord Jesus, and shalt believe in thine heart that God hath raised Him from the dead, thou shalt be saved." Romans 10:9

"For whosoever shall call upon the name of the Lord (Jesus) shall be saved" Romans 10:13

What to pray:

Dear God, I am a sinner, I need forgiveness. I believe that Jesus died and shed His blood for my sins. I am willing to turn from my old life and invite

Jesus into my heart as my savior. Please wash away my sin with the blood of Jesus.